CANCER ETIOLOGY, DIAGNOSIS AND TREATMENTS

UNDERSTANDING A CANCER DIAGNOSIS

CANCER ETIOLOGY, DIAGNOSIS AND TREATMENTS

Additional books and e-books in this series can be found on Nova's website under the Series tab.

Cancer Etiology, Diagnosis and Treatments

Understanding a Cancer Diagnosis

Wellington Pinheiro dos Santos
Maira Araujo de Santana
and
Washington Wagner Azevedo da Silva
Editors

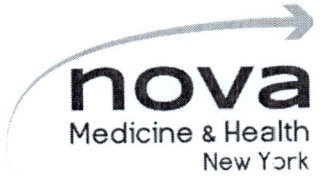

Medicine & Health
New York

Copyright © 2020 by Nova Science Publishers, Inc.

All rights reserved. No part of this book may be reproduced, stored in a retrieval system or transmitted in any form or by any means: electronic, electrostatic, magnetic, tape, mechanical photocopying, recording or otherwise without the written permission of the Publisher.

We have partnered with Copyright Clearance Center to make it easy for you to obtain permissions to reuse content from this publication. Simply navigate to this publication's page on Nova's website and locate the "Get Permission" button below the title description. This button is linked directly to the title's permission page on copyright.com. Alternatively, you can visit copyright.com and search by title, ISBN, or ISSN.

For further questions about using the service on copyright.com, please contact:
Copyright Clearance Center
Phone: +1-(978) 750-8400   Fax: +1-(978) 750-4470   E-mail: info@copyright.com

NOTICE TO THE READER

The Publisher has taken reasonable care in the preparation of this book, but makes no expressed or implied warranty of any kind and assumes no responsibility for any errors or omissions. No liability is assumed for incidental or consequential damages in connection with or arising out of information contained in this book. The Publisher shall not be liable for any special, consequential, or exemplary damages resulting, in whole or in part, from the readers' use of, or reliance upon, this material. Any parts of this book based on government reports are so indicated and copyright is claimed for those parts to the extent applicable to compilations of such works.

Independent verification should be sought for any data, advice or recommendations contained in this book. In addition, no responsibility is assumed by the Publisher for any injury and/or damage to persons or property arising from any methods, products, instructions, ideas or otherwise contained in this publication.

This publication is designed to provide accurate and authoritative information with regard to the subject matter covered herein. It is sold with the clear understanding that the Publisher is not engaged in rendering legal or any other professional services. If legal or any other expert assistance is required, the services of a competent person should be sought. FROM A DECLARATION OF PARTICIPANTS JOINTLY ADOPTED BY A COMMITTEE OF THE AMERICAN BAR ASSOCIATION AND A COMMITTEE OF PUBLISHERS.

Additional color graphics may be available in the e-book version of this book.

Library of Congress Cataloging-in-Publication Data

ISBN: 978-1-53617-520-2
Library of Congress Control Number: 2020932297

Published by Nova Science Publishers, Inc. † New York

CONTENTS

Preface		vii
Acknowledgment		xi
Chapter 1	Considerations of Novel Diagnostic and Therapeutic Approaches to Metastatic Triple-Negative Breast Cancer *Katarzyna Rygiel*	1
Chapter 2	Morphological Decomposition to Detect and Classify Lesions in Mammograms *Sidney Marlon Lopes de Lima,* *Abel Guilhermino da Silva Filho* *and Wellington Pinheiro dos Santos*	27
Chapter 3	Breast Lesions Classification in Frontal Thermographic Images Using Intelligent Systems and Moments of Haralick and Zernike *Maíra Araújo de Santana,* *Jessiane Mônica Silva Pereira,* *Rita de Cássia Fernandes de Lima* *and Wellington Pinheiro dos Santos*	73

Contents

Chapter 4	Lesion Detection in Breast Thermography Using Machine Learning Algorithms without Previous Segmentation *Jessiane Mônica Silva Pereira,* *Maíra Araújo de Santana,* *Rita de Cássia Fernandes de Lima* *and Wellington Pinheiro dos Santos*	**91**
Chapter 5	Dialectical Optimization Method as a Feature Selection Tool for Breast Cancer Diagnosis Using Thermographic Images *Jessiane Mônica Silva Pereira,* *Maíra Araújo de Santana,* *Washington Wagner Azevedo da Silva,* *Rita de Cássia Fernandes de Lima,* *Sidney Marlon Lopes de Lima* *and Wellington Pinheiro dos Santos*	**111**
Chapter 6	Method for Classification of Breast Lesions in Thermographic Images Using ELM Classifiers *Jessiane Mônica Silva Pereira,* *Maíra Araújo de Santana,* *Rita de Cássia Fernandes de Lima,* *Sidney Marlon Lopes de Lima* *and Wellington Pinheiro dos Santos*	**139**

About the Editors   **157**

Index   **159**

PREFACE

"It is a formidable difficulty, and I fear that you ask too much when you expect me to solve it. The past and the present are within the field of my inquiry, but what a man may do in the future is a hard question to answer."

(Sherlock Holmes, in Arthur Conan Doyle's *The Hound of the Baskervilles*)

This phrase is a response from the fictional character Sherlock Holmes to his colleague, Dr Watson, presented in the final chapter, when they are back to Baker Street, London, after solving the case of the Hound of the Baskervilles. In his rich imagination, Sir Arthur Conan Doyle invented stories full of darkness and complexity. Holmes and Watson used to solve these cases by using a creative combination of scientific knowledge, intuition and direct action. These stories populated the minds of generations and continue to influence many fields of arts, like theatre, cinema, literature, and even video games and pop arts.

We are convinced diagnosis can be a deep investigative process, complex by nature. When we face the complexity of diagnosing difficult diseases, specially the several forms of cancer, we are frequently challenged to use not only the plethora of available technologies but, like in Doyle's stories, intuition and direct action. Regarding these available technologies, the diagnostic processes have becoming much more multidisciplinary, demanding the use of an eclectic set of technological methodologies and tools, especially from the Fourth Revolution. Biosensors, Artificial Intelligence, Internet of Things, and 3D Printing have becoming common terms in health research.

Cancer in all its forms has become one of the biggest public health issues of the twentieth century. This phenomenon has been happening worldwide, regardless of the levels of social and economic development of the different nations [1]. Of all types of cancer, breast cancer is the most dangerous for older and middle-aged women, also being the most common form of cancer among female population [1].

Breast cancer is among the five most common cancers worldwide [2]. This disease has been proliferating in both developed and underdeveloped and developing countries. Its incidence rate is increasing with the average life expectancy of the population, and with the adoption of new forms of consumption [1].

Nowadays, there are some preventive strategies for breast cancer, such as stimulating visual inspection and touching of the breasts. However, they are not efficient enough to impact breast cancer mortality rate, since the disease is still being late diagnosed in many cases [1]. For this reason, there is a need to invest in tools for a deeper understanding of the disease, its risk factors, and strategies for early identification and efficient treatment. The existence and availability of these tools in healthcare systems is important, since they may contribute to increase the chances of cure and the treatment options, decreasing mortality rates [1]. Some of these strategies are presented in this book.

Herein this collection book, we present you a set of works from the state-of-the-art dealing with cancer diagnosis using biosensors, artificial intelligence and other approaches.

In the first chapter, called "Considerations of Novel Diagnostic and Therapeutic Approaches to Metastatic Triple-Negative Breast Cancer", Rygiel presents some clinical studies leading to the approval of some innovative targeted therapies and diagnostic strategies for triple-negative breast cancer (TNBC).

Then, in "Morphological Decomposition to detect and classify lesions in mammograms", by Lima, Silva-Filho and Santos, they propose a class of Morphological Decomposition inspired by wavelets to represent regions of interest on mammograms. The approach was combined to artificial intelligence to perform effective breast cancer detection.

In chapter three, "Breast Lesions Classification in Frontal Thermographic Images using Intelligent Systems and Moments of Haralick and Zernike", Santana et al. reached outstanding results using different machine learning approaches to differentiate cystic, malignant and benign lesions in breast thermographic images.

Pereira et al., in "Lesion Detection in Breast Thermography using Machine Learning Algorithms without Previous Segmentation" chapter, achieved excellent performance of machine learning algorithms in detecting the existence of lesions in breast thermography exams.

The fifth chapter, called "Dialectical Optimization Method as a Feature Selection Tool for Breast Cancer Diagnosis using Thermographic Images", by Pereira et al., proposes a features selection model based on the dialectical optimization algorithm (ODM) combined to an Extreme Learning Machine (ELM) as the objective function. This model was applied to the identification of the most relevant features from breast thermographic images, playing an important role in the optimization of computer-aided diagnosis (CAD).

In "Method for Classification of Breast Lesion in Thermographic Images using ELM Classifier", Pereira et al. introduce a method to classify the type of breast lesion in thermographic images using different configurations of Extreme Learning Machines (ELM). This approach has great potential to be used in CAD systems, given the low computational cost associated to ELM.

We hope that the work presented in this collection will show some of the state of the art of innovative techniques based on the Fourth Industrial Revolution to support the diagnosis of cancer, especially breast cancer.

Enjoy your reading!

Prof. Wellington Pinheiro dos Santos, DSc, MSc, EE
Maíra Araújo de Santana, MSc, BSc, BME

December 12, 2019
Recife, Brazil

REFERENCES

[1] Groot, M. T., Baltussen, R., Uyl-de Groot, C. A., Anderson, B. O., and Hortobágyi, G. N. 2006. "Costs and health effects of breast cancer interventions in epidemiologically different regions of Africa, North America, and Asia." *The Breast Journal* 12(s1):S81-S90.

[2] Shrivastava, S. R., Shrivastava, P. S., and Jegadeesh, R. 2017. "Ensuring early detection of cancer in low- and middle-income nations: World health organization." *Archives of Medicine and Health Sciences* 5(1):141.

ACKNOWLEDGMENTS

We are grateful to our families, friends, and colleagues from the Research Groupe of Biomedical Computing of the Federal University of Pernambuco, Recife, Brazil, for their support in several stages of this work, especially for the elaboration of the chapters on the use of machine learning to aid breast cancer diagnosis.

We would like to thank the Brazilian research agencies CAPES, CNPq and FACEPE, for the partial support of the researches presented in this book.

Last but not least, we also thank the authors for their kind contributions for this collection.

In: Understanding a Cancer Diagnosis
Editors: W. P. dos Santos et al.
ISBN: 978-1-53617-520-2
© 2020 Nova Science Publishers, Inc.

Chapter 1

CONSIDERATIONS OF NOVEL DIAGNOSTIC AND THERAPEUTIC APPROACHES TO METASTATIC TRIPLE-NEGATIVE BREAST CANCER

Katarzyna Rygiel[*]

Department of Family Practice,
Medical University of Silesia (SUM), Zabrze, Poland

ABSTRACT

Traditionally, breast cancer (BC) was classified into different histological subtypes, mostly on the basis of microscopic and immunohistochemical (IHC) assessment. With the advent of personalized medicine, a better understanding of the carcinogenesis process and tumor biology has led to the discovery of novel, targeted diagnostic and therapeutic approaches. Recently, some new management options have emerged in the field of metastatic BC, transforming the course of this disease and improving the patient quality of life

---

[*] Corresponding Author's Email: kasiaalpha@yahoo.co.uk

However, these options are still very limited for triple-negative breast cancer (TNBC). Nevertheless, the remarkable progress of knowledge relevant to the TNBC complex biology, as well as the discovery of some innovative molecular targets, have expanded the horizons of care for women with metastatic TNBC. In fact, TNBC is a heterogeneous disease, involving various subtypes of breast cancer (BC). TNBC is estrogen receptor (ER)-negative, progesterone receptor (PR)-negative, and human epidermal growth factor receptor 2 (HER2)-negative. In addition, androgen receptor (AR) is expressed in approximately 10% - 32% of TNBC. In general, TNBC is characterized by worst outcomes, such as higher risks of relapse and visceral crisis compared to other BC subtypes. It has been estimated that TNBC represents about 60% of cases in patients with a *BRCA1* mutation and 20% in *BRCA2* mutation carriers. Because of scarce treatment options for TNBC, there is a necessity to develop innovative diagnostic and therapeutic approaches for patients with TNBC. In response to this challenge, various strategies (e.g., poly(ADP-ribose) polymerase (PARP) inhibitors, immunotherapy, and androgen receptor (AR) inhibitors) have been investigated in clinical trials, aiming to match such therapies with the specific TNBC subtypes. In order to properly stratify patients to these novel therapies, a precise diagnostic workup has to be performed.

This chapter presents some diagnostic considerations related to women with locally advanced or metastatic TNBC and *BRCA1/2* mutations. It discusses the clinical studies leading to the approval of some innovative targeted therapies for TNBC and emphasizes the key implications for further research and medical practice. Moreover, this chapter addresses patient education and engagement that are crucial for a successful management process, and the improvement of disease outcomes, and patient quality of life.

Keywords: Triple-Negative Breast Cancer (TNBC), *BRCA1/2* mutation, targeted therapy, poly(ADP-ribose) polymerase (PARP) inhibitors, programmed cell death protein-1 (PD-1), programmed cell death ligand 1 (PD-L1), checkpoint inhibitors, androgen receptor (AR) inhibitors

INTRODUCTION

Breast cancer (BC) represents the most common neoplastic disease and the second leading cause of mortality among women worldwide [1]. In the past, BC was classified into different histological subtypes, mostly on the basis of microscopic and immunohistochemical (IHC) evaluation of hormone receptors (HRs) and human epidermal growth factor 2.

Triple-Negative Breast Cancer (TNBC) is a very difficult-to-treat, heterogeneous malignancy, involving various subtypes (Figure 1) that account for almost 20% of all BCs [2]. TNBC is characterized by estrogen receptor (ER)-negative, progesterone receptor (PR)-negative, and human epidermal growth factor receptor 2 (HER2)-negative status [2]. Moreover, androgen receptor (AR) is expressed in about 10% - 32% of TNBC [3]. Unfortunately, TNBC has a very poor prognosis (e.g., elevated risks of relapse and visceral crisis) compared to other BC subtypes [4]. TNBC represents approximately 60% of cases in women with a *BRCA1* mutation, and 20% in a *BRCA2* mutation carriers [5].

BRCA1 and *BRCA2* represent tumor suppressor genes that play a key role in repairing DNA damages in the cells [6]. It should be highlighted that TNBC is the predominant subtype of BC among women, who harbor a germline *BRCA* mutation [7]. Since treatment options for TNBC are very scarce (e.g., cytotoxic chemotherapy (CHT)) there is a necessity to develop novel therapeutic options, associated with reliable diagnostic tests. With the development of precision medicine, current progress in molecular profiling and genomic sequencing allowed a better understanding of metastatic BC progression [8]. Hopefully, these new insights into the molecular mechanisms of various TNBC subtypes can also lead to the development of novel diagnostic tests, which will be crucial for the most accurate selecting patients for novel targeted therapies.

This chapter presents some important diagnostic considerations related to patients with locally advanced or metastatic TNBC. It summarizes the clinical studies on some promising, innovative treatments for patients with TNBC (e.g., poly(ADP-ribose) polymerase (PARP) inhibitors, immunotherapy, and androgen receptor (AR) inhibitors) and underscores implications for further research and medical practice.

In addition, this chapter addresses key aspects of patient education and engagement that are essential for a successful management process, aimed at improving not only the disease outcomes but also the patient's functional condition and quality of life.

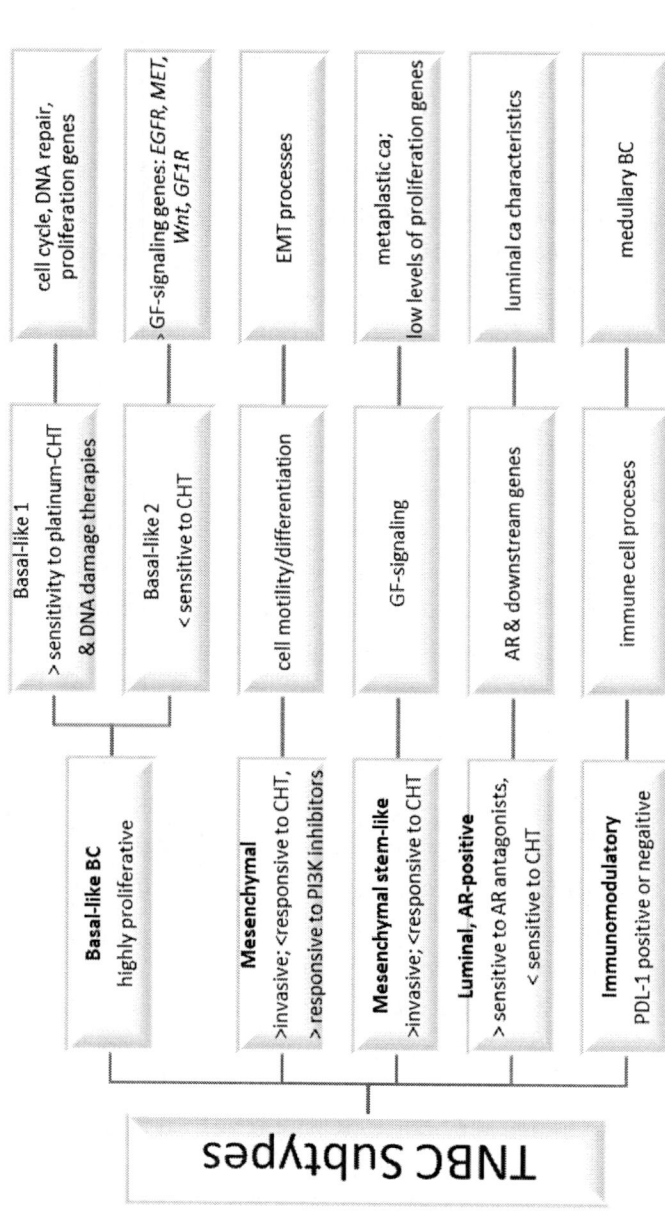

Figure 1. Subtypes of TNBC and their main signaling pathways.
[Abbreviations: AR, androgen receptor; BC, breast cancer; ca, cancer; EMT, epithelial–mesenchymal transition; CHT, chemotherapy; PDL-1, programmed death ligand 1; PI3K, phosphoinositide 3-kinase; TNBC, Triple-Negative Breast Cancer; GF, growth factor].

CORRELATIONS OF GERMLINE *BRCA* MUTATIONS WITH TNBC – TAKING ADVANTAGE OF "VULNERABLE" TUMORS

Despite unquestionable therapeutic advances in the field of BC, TNBC still remains an unmet medical need. This is partially due to the fact that TNBC has a very high potential for biological changes during the disease course. The current progress in tumor sequencing methodologies has contributed to the identification of molecular targets and pathways involved in the carcinogenesis and metastatic progression of BC [9]. Recently, TNBC has been classified into five categories, which correspond with distinct therapeutic sensitivities (Figure 1) [2, 10]. *BRCA1* and *BRCA2* genes play a key role in repairing double-strand DNA injuries [7]. The *BRCA1* mutations are mostly associated with TNBC, and the *BRCA2* mutations can be related to HR-positive/HER2-negative BC [7].

The term "BRCAness" was created to characterize the tumors, which are BRCA-proficient, but behave as if they were deficient in DNA double-strand break repair (via homologous recombination) [11]. In addition, some similar defects in homologous recombination mechanism may occur after the methylation of *BRCA* gene promoter and the alteration of some other genes, such as TP53, PALB2, and ATM [11]. Tumors harboring defects in *BRCA1/2* genes (resulting in an inability to repair the double-strand DNA breaks) are sensitive to the blockage of single-strand DNA repair [12]. The poly (ADP-ribose) polymerase (PARP) inhibitors are targeted agents that have recently been approved for the treatment of metastatic TNBC with *BRCA1/2* mutations [12]. It should be noted that in patients with TNBC, the BRCAness phenotype can be related not only to *BRCA* mutations but also to *BRCA1* promoter methylation or low *BRCA1* mRNA or protein expression [7, 12].

Table 1. Selected clinical trials of PARP inhibitors, immune checkpoint inhibitors, and AR inhibitors in patients with advanced or metastatic triple negative breast cancer

Clinical trial phase, identifier	Therapeutic agent/class, dose	Trial endpoints	Practical implications of the trial	Ref.
OlympiAD, phase III NCT02000622	Olaparib PARP inhibitor 300 mg bid PO	OS, AEs	efficacy & safety of olaparib vs. CHT of physician's choice (capecitabine, vinorelbine, or eribulin) in patients with a gBRCA mutation and HER2-negative metastatic BC; possible OS benefit with olaparib, in patients who did not receive CHT for metastatic BC; good tolerability of olaparib	[14, 15]
EMBRACA phase III NCT01945775	Talazoparib PARP inhibitor 1 mg qd PO	PFS	efficacy & safety of talazoparib vs. CHT of physician's choice (capecitabine, eribulin, gemcitabine or vinorelbine) in patients with gBRCA mutation, HER2-negative locally advanced or metastatic BC; improved median PFS in the talazoparib group	[16]
IMpassion130 phase III NCT02425891	Atezolizumab anti-PD-L1 antibody	PFS	atezolizumab with nab-paclitaxel vs. placebo with nab-paclitaxel for patients with previously untreated advanced or metastatic TNBC; PFS and OS were improved in PD-L1–positive patients; the PD-L1 expression in immune cells is a predictor of response; in PD-L1–negative patients, there was no therapeutic effect of atezolizumab and nab-paclitaxel	[17]
TONIC phase II NCT02499367	Nivolumab anti-PD-1 antibody	PFS	stimulation of the anticancer immune responses (by induction treatment with RT or CHT) to make the tumor microenvironment more susceptible to nivolumab in metastatic TNBC; short term induction with RT or low dose CHT (e.g., doxorubicin, cyclophosphamide, or cisplatin) before nivolumab is feasible in metastatic TNBC	[18]
KEYNOTE-119 (ongoing) phase III NCT02555657	Pembrolizumab anti-PD-1 antibody	PFS, OS	pembrolizumab alone vs. single-agent CHT of physician's choice in patients with locally advanced or metastatic TNBC	[19]

Clinical trial phase, identifier	Therapeutic agent/class, dose	Trial endpoints	Practical implications of the trial	Ref.
KEYNOTE-086 phase II NCT02447003	Pembrolizumab anti-PD-1 antibody	ORR, safety	pembrolizumab monotherapy - a manageable safety profile & durable antitumor activity as first-line therapy for patients with PD-L1-positive metastatic TNBC	[20]
A phase II trial NCT00468715	Bicalutamide AR inhibitor 150 mg qd PO	CBR at 6 months	bicalutamide for the treatment of patients with AR-positive, ER-negative, PR-negative metastatic BC	[23]
UCBG 12-1 phase II NCT01842321	Abiraterone AR inhibitor 160 mg qd PO	CBR at 6 months	abiraterone plus prednisone in patients with AR-positive locally advanced or metastatic TNBC	[24]
A phase II trial NCT01889238	Enzalutamide AR inhibitor 160 mg qd PO	CBR at 16 weeks	[+] clinical activity & safety of enzalutamide in patients with advanced or metastatic AR-positive TNBC	[25]
ENDEAR (ongoing) phase III NCT02677896	Enzalutamide AR inhibitor 160 mg qd PO	PFS	the efficacy & safety of enzalutamide, as monotherapy or in combination with paclitaxel CHT, in patients with locally advanced or metastatic TNBC; PREDICT-AR -a novel diagnostic assay used to enroll patients with AR-positive TNBC	[26]

Abbreviations: AEs, adverse events; BC, breast cancer; HER2, human epidermal growth factor receptor 2; ER, estrogen receptor; HR, hormone receptor; PR, progesterone receptor; gBRCAm, germline BRCA-mutation; CBR, clinical benefit rate; CHT, chemotherapy; m, metastatic; PARP, poly (ADP-ribose) polymerase; PD-1, programmed cell death protein-1; PD-L1, programmed death ligand 1; IHC, immunohistochemistry; OS, overall survival; PFS, progression-free survival, ORR, overall response rate; RT, radiation therapy; TNBC, triple negative breast cancer; vs., versus, PO, orally; bid, twice daily; qd, once daily.

According to a recent TNT trial, in women with metastatic TNBC (with changes in DNA repair, which were similar to those of *BRCA*-mutated tumors), half of the patients were treated with carboplatin, and the other half with docetaxel [13]. It has been determined that in this unselected group, carboplatin and docetaxel revealed similar efficacy [13]. However, it should be highlighted that in patients with g*BRCA* mutation, carboplatin doubled the response rate, compared to the one from the docetaxel group (68% vs. 33%) [13].

In the OlympiAD trial, which included patients with g*BRCA* mutated metastatic TNBC, olaparib (a PARP inhibitor) was compared with CHT (not platinum-based) (Table 1) [14, 15]. The OlympiAD trial revealed an improvement in median PFS (7 versus 4.2 months) and ORR from 28.8 to 59.9% [14, 15]. Similarly, in the EMBRACA trial, in patients with advanced BC and a g*BRCA* mutation, talazoparib (a PARP inhibitor) has revealed a better median PFS, compared with non-platinum-based CHT (8.6 vs. 5.6 months), and an improvement in ORR (from 27.7 to 62.2%) (Table 1) [16]. At this point, it would be merited to directly compare platinum-based CHT with PARP inhibitors, in women with g*BRCA* mutated tumors.

MUTATIONS IN *BRCA* GENES AND PD-L1–EXPRESSION ON THE IMMUNE CELLS - AS INDEPENDENT BIOMARKERS IN PATIENTS WITH TNBC

An association between the tumor biology, immune cells, and the *BRCA1/2* mutation status was studied in a clinical trial, which investigated benefits from combination therapy, including atezolizumab and nab-paclitaxel (Table 1) [17]. It has been revealed that among patients with CD8+ T cells on their tumors, clinical benefits, in terms of PFS and OS, were noted only if these tumors were also PD-L1 immune cell-positive [17]. In particular, in patients who were positive for both CD8+ expression and PD-L1 immune cell expression, significant clinical benefits were observed (e.g., PFS and OS) from the combination therapy [17]. However, patients whose tumors contained stromal tumor infiltrating lymphocytes (TILs) and PD-L1-negative expression on the immune cells had no benefits from the addition of atezolizumab [17]. In addition, patients whose tumors had stromal TILs and PD-L1-positive expression on the immune cells had also a significant improvement in PFS and OS from the use of atezolizumab plus nab-paclitaxel combined therapy [17].

It should be highlighted that among patients with *BRCA1/2* mutated tumors, a significant improvement in PFS was observed, with the use of this combination therapy, only if their tumors were also PD-L1 immune cell-positive [17]. These data may indicate that mutations in *BRCA* genes and PD-L1–expressing immune cells represent independent biomarkers. In fact, in the IMpassion130 trial, approximately 15% of patients had *BRCA* mutations [17]. Among them, no relations between treatment and survival advantages were found in the PD-L1–negative subgroup. In contrast, *BRCA* mutation–positive and PD-L1–positive status were significantly correlated with PFS benefits from the immunotherapy and CHT combination [17]. IMpassion130 trial, as a positive study on immunotherapy in the TNBC setting, represents a step forward, bringing new hope to both patients and their medical providers [17].

In the TONIC trial, strategies stimulating the anticancer immune responses (by induction treatment with radiotherapy (RT) or CHT) in order to make the tumor microenvironment more susceptible to nivolumab (an anti-PD-1 antibody), in metastatic TNBC were investigated (Table 1) [18]. Findings of the TONIC study have shown that the short term induction with RT or low dose CHT (e.g., doxorubicin, cyclophosphamide, or cisplatin) before administration of nivolumab is feasible in metastatic TNBC [18]. In addition, the recent KEYNOTE-119 and KEYNOTE-086 trials, exploring pembrolizumab (an anti-PD-1 antibody) have revealed a manageable safety profile and durable antitumor activity of this agent (as first-line therapy), among patients with PD-L1-positive metastatic TNBC (Table 1) [19, 20].

ANDROGEN SIGNALING PATHWAY IN TNBC

Since novel treatment approaches are necessary for TNBC, the androgen signaling has been explored in details in this subtype of BC. It should be noted that androgen receptor (AR) expression in TNBC is variable (e.g., 10% has been accepted as a cutoff point for AR positivity in nuclear staining), depending on the testing methods, cutoff values for positivity, and individual tumor characteristics [21]. However, it has been suggested that there is a correlation between a higher level of AR expression and better patient outcomes. Therefore, women with AR-dependent TNBCs can have a better prognosis compared to those with not AR-dependent TNBCs [21]. For instance, a luminal AR subtype of TNBC, which is dependent on AR signaling has been identified, and AR was assessed as a possible target in advanced TNBC [22]. Recent clinical trials have indicated that there are some clinical benefits related to the AR inhibition in the metastatic BC setting (Table 1) [23]. In particular, an AR inhibitor, bicalutamide, has revealed a signal of activity and acceptable tolerability, in a subset of patients with BC (whose tumors tested greater than 10% AR-positive), who were conventionally treated with cytotoxic CHT [23]. AR was expressed in 12% of patients with ER/PR-negative BC screened for this trial. The clinical benefit rate (CBR) of 19% observed with bicalutamide has revealed the efficacy of androgen blockade in a select group of women with ER/PR-negative, AR-positive BC [23]. Subsequently, abiraterone (a 17 alphahydroxylase inhibitor), has been explored in patients with advanced or metastatic TNBC (Table 1) [24]. In this study, abiraterone was associated with a CBR of 20% at 6 months, an ORR of 6.7%, and a mPFS of 2.8 months [24].

The efficacy and safety of another AR inhibitor, enzalutamide, was investigated in a clinical trial that involved patients with locally advanced or metastatic AR-positive TNBC (Table 1) [25]. In this study, a higher rate of AR positivity could have been attributed to the lower AR expression cutoff values and improvement of immunohistochemistry (IHC) techniques [25]. The primary outcome was CBR at 16 weeks, and the secondary outcomes included CBR at 24 weeks, progression-free survival (PFS), and adverse effects [25]. More than half of the study patients received therapy with enzalutamide, resulting in CBRs of 25% at 16 weeks and 20% at 24 weeks [25]. Subsequently, the CBRs were improved to 35% at 16 weeks and 29% at 24 weeks (e.g., with AR positivity above 10%) [25]. In addition, the median progression-free survival (mPFS) rates were 14.7 weeks in women with tumors, which harbored an AR positivity of at least 10%, and 12.6 weeks in women, whose tumors had AR positivity in the range from 0 to 10% [25]. Median overall survival (mOS) was 12.7 months in the entire study population and 17.6 months in the subgroup with AR positivity of at least 10% [25]. Fatigue was the main treatment-related adverse event (e.g., grade 3 or higher with an incidence of above 2%.) [25]. Overall, enzalutamide has shown some beneficial activity and acceptable safety profile, in patients with advanced or metastatic AR-positive TNBC [25]. Furthermore, a predictive gene expression classifier test, Predict-AR, was able to more accurately distinguish responsive patients in the whole study population [25]. For instance, CBR at 24 weeks in Predict-AR-positive patients was 36%, compared to 6% among those, whose tumors were Predict-AR-negative [25]. Moreover, PFS rates were 16 weeks in women with Predict-AR-positive TNBC and 8 weeks in Predict-AR-negative patients [25].

The ongoing ENDEAR study is assessing the efficacy and safety of enzalutamide, as monotherapy or in combination with paclitaxel CHT, among women with locally advanced or metastatic TNBC. Moreover, the ENDEAR trial explores a novel genomic diagnostic assay, PREDICT-AR, which is based on RNA expression profile [26]. The PREDICT-AR test can be superior to the AR staining for the prediction of benefits from enzalutamide. This assay is not yet the standard of care. However, in the near future, it may become a new diagnostic strategy to enroll patients with AR-positive TNBC to clinical studies assessing effects of enzalutamide [26]. In spite of many positive results revealed among a well-selected patients, AR inhibitors are not yet recommended as the standard of care, pending further trials that will determine more precise prognostic and predictive biomarkers [27].

PATIENT-CENTERED EDUCATION ABOUT SELECTED DIAGNOSTIC AND THERAPEUTIC STRATEGIES FOR TNBC

Even though TNBC constitutes fewer than 20% of all BCs, it is responsible for disproportionate BC morbidity and mortality, especially in young women [28]. This "scary" information often has a deeply negative impact on the psychophysical condition of many females, who have been diagnosed with TNBC. However, the good news is that recently, several research studies have shown that women with TNBC can have a better response to conventional CHT than women with other BC types [29]. In addition, currently, there are some new promising, approved or emerging therapies for TNBC, even in the metastatic stage. Nevertheless, such positive messages can often be overlooked or misunderstood by the overwhelmed TNBC patients. It should be highlighted that the key to a meaningful, reassuring conversation with patients is the explicit statement that TNBC is treatable and can have a good outcome. Therefore, physicians and other MDT members should explain, in simple terms, the implications of TNBC diagnosis and treatment to their patients.

In order to help physicians effectively communicate with such patients, certain instructive patterns are necessary. Since women with TNBC are usually very worried about their "terrible "diagnosis, they require, in addition to a comprehensive medical therapy, a lot of education, empowerment, support, and reassurance (Figure 2). Unfortunately, a diagnosis of TNBC typically generates feelings of anxiety, fear, sadness, depression, and hopelessness. For instance, at the time of diagnosis, some women may perceive TNBC as a "death sentence." They may have an impression that there is no reason to even start treatment since this is an incurable type of cancer. At this point, a straight-forward, professional conversation about how TNBC can be managed is crucial to reverse this detrimental way of thinking. In fact, only a few patients correctly understand the concept of TNBC. Therefore, it is necessary to tell the patients that TNBC is currently treatable, and it is worthwhile to participate in available clinical trials, which may offer some additional, promising options. In essence, the physicians should skillfully translate the diagnosis of TNBC for their patients. This requires explaining to a patient some key points about TNBC biology and the management options. For instance, it is appropriate to tell the patient that TNBC is a type of BC, which does not respond to endocrine therapy or anti-HER2-targeted therapy, but due to its rapid growth, it may positively respond to CHT [13]. Moreover, in the metastatic TNBC setting, a physician should point out that the considered CHT will have tolerable side effects. During an open dialogue with the patient, the physician should discuss all the appropriate treatment options, including possible participation in available clinical trials [19, 26]. Also, it is imperative to explain that not all cases of TNBC are the same. Since TNBC is a heterogeneous disease, there is only a subgroup of patients with TNBC that progresses rapidly and can be resistant to CHT. Furthermore, it should be underscored that this subset of TNBC can be responsive to some novel, targeted therapies, characterized by low toxicity and convenient, oral form of administration [14-20]. At the beginning of the educational consultation with a patient, it is worthwhile to describe a whole spectrum of BC, and adequately position TNBC within that spectrum. Also, the concept of early vs. late BC stage is a perspective, which should be presented, when explaining TNBC to the patients.

The next key area for patient education is BC biology. For instance, the physician should explain that slowly-growing tumors are not going to respond to aggressive CHT, and are related to a risk of recurrence (e.g., in the next 10-20 years). In contrast, in the case of TNBC, it is more probable that the recurrence will occur within the first 3-5 years after diagnosis. However, the well-selected CHT or targeted therapy can more likely bring clinical advantages, depending on tumor biology. Therefore, TNBC should be viewed more positively, since it can be effectively treated with CHT or novel targeted therapies [13-20]. Furthermore, any women, who are undergoing TNBC treatment should at least consider participation in available clinical trials [19, 26]. At this point, some convenient online options, organized in collaboration with the National Cancer Institute, matching patients with available trials should be assessed (Figure 3).

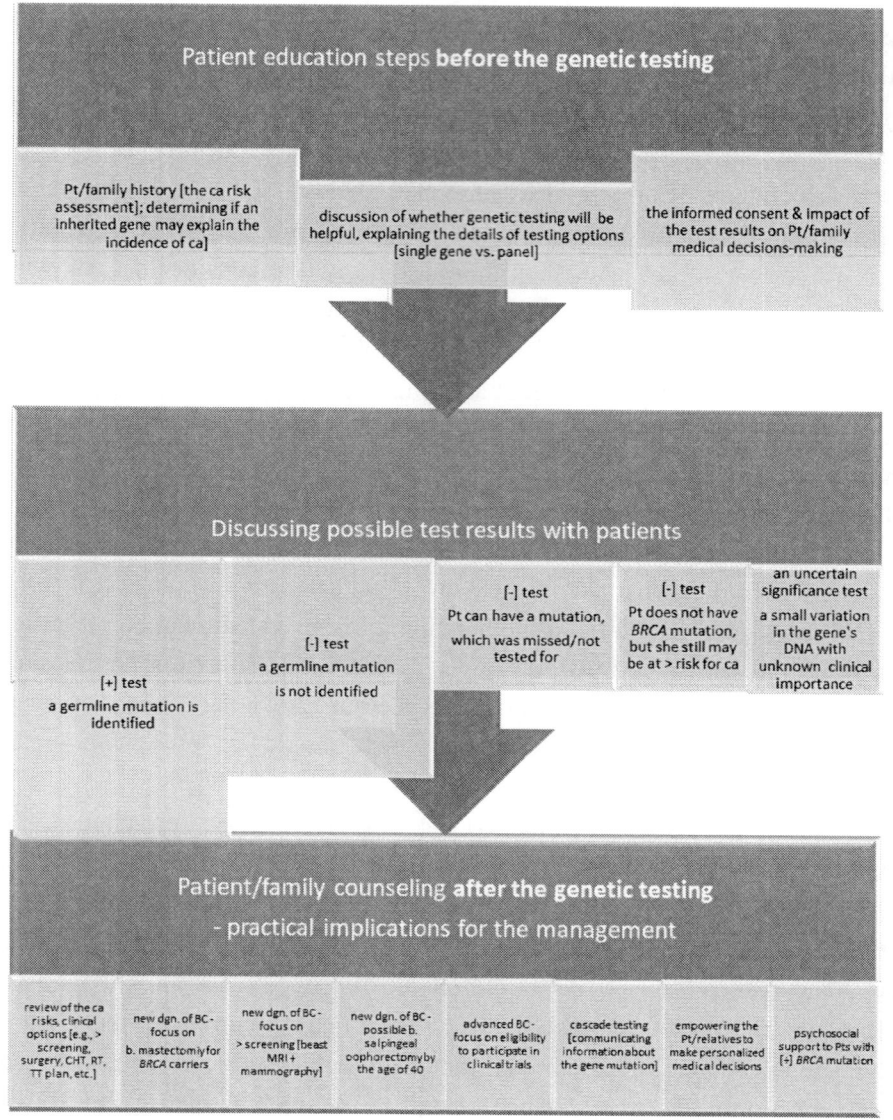

Figure 2. A sequence of BC patient education and *BRCA* genetic testing.
[Abbreviations: b., bilateral; BC, breast cancer; ca, cancer; CHT, chemotherapy; dgn., diagnosis; RT, radiation therapy; TT, targeted therapy; Pt, patient; PARP, poly (ADP-ribose) polymerase].

Considerations of Novel Diagnostic and Therapeutic Approaches ... 15

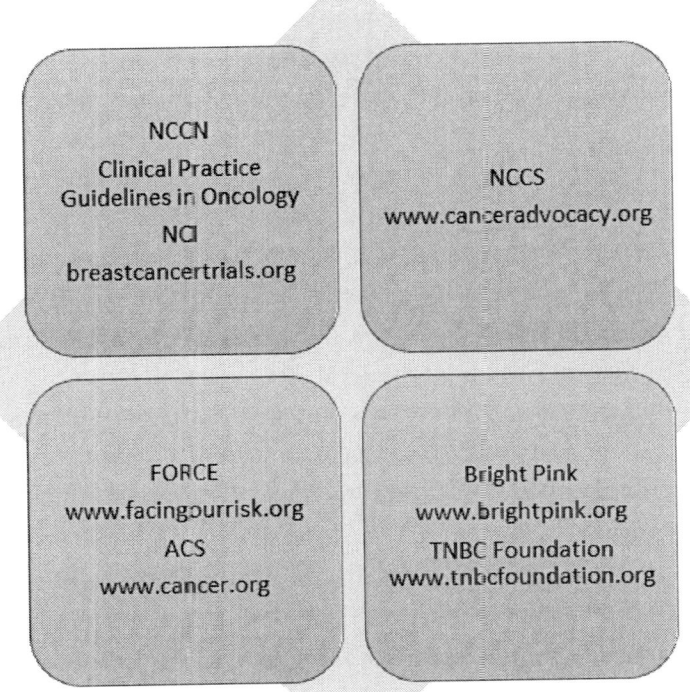

Figure 3. Helpful management resources for physicians and TNBC patients. [Abbreviations: ACS, American Cancer Society; BC, breast cancer; NCCN, National Comprehensive Cancer Network; NCCS, National Coalition for Cancer Survivorship; NCI, National Cancer Institute; FORCE, Facing Our Risk of Cancer Empowerment; TNBC, Triple Negative Breast Cancer Foundation].

In addition, it is helpful to inquire what approaches are currently being explored to improve TNBC outcomes. For instance, the National Comprehensive Cancer Network (NCCN) issues recommendations for the standard treatments of TNBC. In practical terms, it is convenient to use the NCCN guidelines, so that physicians can discuss in details the standard treatment options with their patients. Application of these types of tools plays an important role in empowering of the women with TNBC and their family members (who may also be upset and confused by the TNBC diagnosis).

Another problem is that the patient with a diagnosis of TNBC may be exposed to a great deal of misinformation from some unprofessional sources (e.g., aggressive pseudo-medical advertisement, family members or friends). Even in the case of advanced and metastatic TNBC, some reasonable treatment options exist. The most helpful approach for patients is to provide them with as much practical education as possible before they initiate their oncology management. In general, it is more beneficial for the women to take the time to carefully consider all the therapeutic options, rather than to "rush" into the first presented treatment, due to anxiety. Also, it should be reiterated that not all TNBCs are the same. Some patients may respond to different therapies for a year or longer in the metastatic setting. In contrast, some other patients may have cancers that progress rapidly. In general, both physicians and patients should not make premature assumptions about how a tumor will respond to CHT until treatment starts and the results can be assessed.

GERMLINE *BRCA1/2* MUTATION AND BC RISK - TESTING CRITERIA AND TREATMENT DECISION-MAKING

It has been estimated that approximately 5%-10% of BCs are associated with inherited genetic mutations, such as *BRCA1* and *BRCA2* [30]. Figure 4 presents the main reasons for genetic testing for *BRCA* mutation among BC patients. Such patients and their family members need to be clearly informed of why someone should undergo genetic testing for *BRCA*. In particular, it should be pointed out that this testing helps identify the cause of BC in an individual woman or her family. Moreover, it allows a more accurate cancer risk evaluation, as well as an individualized screening and prevention patterns. Also, such testing may provide an opportunity to participate in novel targeted therapies (e.g., PARP inhibitors). In general, candidates for *BRCA* testing can be divided into three 3 groups, including 1) women who are concerned, since they have a family history and wish to know if there is a genetic cause of their cancer, 2) women with a history of BC, who were not tested at the time, when they were diagnosed, but presently, are concerned about their relatives, or about a potential risk for another cancer (e.g., contralateral BC or ovarian cancer), 3) women with a recent diagnosis of BC, who want to make the most optimal treatment decisions. In addition, age is very important for consideration of genetic testing at BC diagnosis, and it should be underscored that women who are diagnosed at a young age should undergo *BRCA* testing. Specific *BRCA1/2* testing criteria are presented in reference 31. Moreover, patients should know that their test results can have implications for their close relatives.

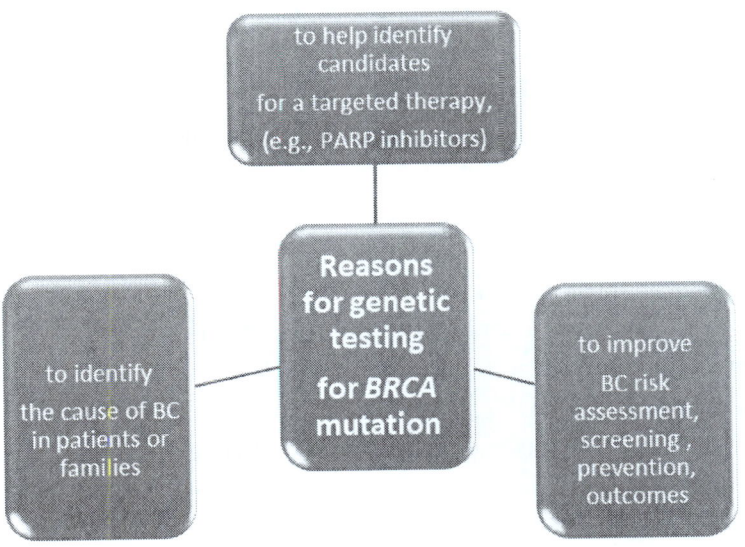

Figure 4. Main reasons for genetic testing for BRCA mutation among BC patients. [Abbreviations: BC, breast cancer; PARP, poly (ADP-ribose) polymerase].

GENETIC COUNSELING ABOUT *BRCA1/2* MUTATIONS FROM THE PATIENT'S PERSPECTIVE

Patient education about genetic testing should include a thorough discussion of risks, available options, and implications (Figure 2), with follow-up sessions in the multidisciplinary setting. It should be highlighted that genetic counseling is always initiated by taking a personal and family history that is subsequently used to appraise the cancer risk. The genetic expert attempts to determine if there is an inherited gene, which may explain the incidence of cancer in the family. If there is a high probability that genetic testing could be helpful, then the consultation focuses on the most suitable options for genetic testing. Moreover, the discussion about the possible test results should be conducted before scheduling and after obtaining these findings (Figure 3). This is mostly because many patients believe that the test results will be positive for the *BRCA1/2* mutation or negative (absence of the *BRCA1/2* mutation). When the *BRCA1/2* mutation has been identified, the recommendations will indicate how to manage the patient, step by step (e.g., surgery, CHT, targeted therapy, or enhanced screening procedures) (Figure 2).

When a *BRCA1/2* mutation has not been identified (a negative test result) can indicate that this person does not have a mutation. Nevertheless, such a person may still have an increased risk for cancer, due to some other factors. Also, the interpretation of negative test results may be difficult, since the applied methodology might have missed the mutation. In addition to positive or negative test result options, there is a third possibility, which is a variant of uncertain significance (e.g., the laboratory identifies a small variation in the gene's DNA, but is unable to determine if this is clinically important). Both patients and physicians need to be prepared ahead of time to cope with the relevant frustration in a calm manner (Figure 2). It should be highlighted that the genetic counseling session needs to be conducted in a very structured way, for a patient with newly diagnosed BC, who is focused on starting the treatment process. Furthermore, the counseling approach needs to be individualized in the case of a patient with advanced or metastatic BC, who is considering genetic testing to determine, if she may be eligible for participation in a clinical study (e.g., for therapy with PARP inhibitors). At this point, the counseling should be focused on patients' individual clinical scenario and personal preferences, to help with the most appropriate decision-making (Figure 2).

Continuation of patient education after genetic testing is extremely important and should be conducted by a multidisciplinary team (MDT). In particular, patients who have a *BRCA1* or *BRCA2* mutation should undergo a detailed consultation with a genetic specialist, medical oncologist, surgeon, psychologist, and nurse. The MDT should discuss various medical options (e.g., enhanced screening, types of surgery, CHT, or targeted therapy) and the relevant risks (Figure 2). It is crucial to help the newly diagnosed patient to prepare for the next step of her management. Many issues require clarification, like, for instance, increased risk for cancer in the other breast. In fact, only the women who carry a *BRCA* mutation are at elevated risk of contralateral BC. Moreover, the woman's and engagement in her own care are essential for adherence to medical advice, and self-care. Such empowered patients should stay motivated and behave like partners in their professional relationship with MDT members. For instance, there is an option of choosing bilateral mastectomies for patients, who are *BRCA* carriers and have a 60% risk of a contralateral BC. However, it should be pointed out that such a prophylactic mastectomy is not necessary. For the women, who select the prophylactic mastectomy, there is now the possibility of performing a nipple-sparing surgery, which can be more suitable than the previous standard technique. Furthermore, when the newly diagnosed patient does not choose mastectomy, then the counseling is focused on regular, enhanced screening (e.g., adding breast MRI to yearly mammography) (Figure 2) [31]. Ovarian cancer risk is another important topic of discussion. In particular, *BRCA* carriers should be recommended to have bilateral salpingeal oophorectomy by the age of 40 years [31].

In addition to direct interaction with BC patients, implications of genetic counseling involve some difficult tasks related to the "cascade testing." This means informing the patient's relatives about the presence of gene mutation that needs to be effectively communicated to family members, who may have elevated cancer risk (Figure 2). In a consequence, testing can be advised for some relatives, in order to improve their knowledge and ability to make informed decisions for individual medical management. Since this situation often creates a lot of anxiety, psychological and social support needs to be provided for patients and their relatives on a regular basis, as well as updated resources for physicians (Figure 3). In addition to just information about the disease, organizations such as the American Cancer

Society (ACS) and the Triple Negative Breast Cancer Foundation can offer connection with support groups (e.g., available online or in local communities). Sharing information will allow patients and their family members to be better equipped and resilient when facing many challenges related to TNBC.

DIRECTIONS FOR FURTHER RESEARCH ON SELECTED DIAGNOSTIC AND THERAPEUTIC ISSUES IN TNBC

Due to rapid progress in molecular characteristics of TNBC, many modern therapeutics, including PARP inhibitors, immune checkpoint inhibitors, androgen receptor (AR) inhibitors, antibody-drug conjugates, and tyrosine kinase inhibitors are being explored for this highly aggressive subtype of BC [32]. It is crucial to properly identify patients, who may favorably respond to such therapies. Moreover, in the dynamic interactions between the cancer cells and various types of immune system cells, reliable biomarkers are needed, in order to more precisely predict the effects of the novel therapeutics in patients with TNBC. Such biomarkers should include the *BRCA1/2* mutation status, PD-1/PD-L1 status, and tumor mutational burden/load [32, 33].

Further studies in patients with TNBC should explore predictive and prognostic biomarkers for proper stratification of patients, who would be the most appropriate candidates for these novel therapies [32, 33]. Moreover, the optimal timing of administration and the best therapeutic modalities (e.g., CHT, immunotherapy, targeted therapy or RT, administered as monotherapy or in combination, as well as their appropriate sequences) represent some unanswered questions, which need to be addressed by future trials [32, 33, 34]. It should be noted that the majority of clinical trials have been conducted in unselected TNBC populations, looking for signals of efficacy during subgroup analyses. However, in the future, prospective, biomarker-based approaches are needed, for the development of targeted therapies. In particular, long-term survival outcomes, clinical efficacy, safety, and tolerability issues have to be investigated in large-scale trials, in women with TNBC [35]

CONCLUSION

TNBC, as a heterogeneous disease with various molecular and biologic subtypes, is very challenging to treat. In fact, TNBC is characterized by higher rates of relapse, greater metastatic potential, and shorter overall survival (OS), compared with other BC subtypes. However, recent diagnostic advances enable much more precise tumor characterization, providing details that can be subsequently integrated with clinical and histopathological data. This, in turn, can facilitate risk stratification of patients, guide treatment decisions, and improve surveillance. At present, some innovative therapies, for specific molecular targets, have contributed to significant improvements in the clinical outcomes, among women with TNBC. In particular, PARP inhibitors (e.g., in germline *BRCA1/2* carriers) and immune-checkpoint inhibitions (e.g., in cases of tumors with PD-L1–positive expression on the immune cells) have recently been approved as targeted treatments. This is very optimistic for both patients with TNBC and their clinicians.

The new insights into the molecular mechanisms of different TNBC subtypes have contributed to the development of innovative therapies, such as PARP inhibitors, AR inhibitors, and immunotherapy with checkpoint inhibitors. It should be highlighted that molecular diagnostic tests are crucial for the most appropriate selecting patients for these targeted therapies. It should be noted that precision medicine is gradually arriving at the bedside of women with TNBC. However, medical teams (in both clinical and research settings) are facing many challenges, such as finding the most accurate biomarkers for prediction of response or resistance to particular therapies, and the right sequence or combination of available treatments. Simultaneously, these complex medical issues need to be explained to patients with TNBC, in a simple, clear, and practical manner, so that they can feel comfortable, and behave as knowledgeable, empowered, and fully engaged partners in their own comprehensive medical care.

REFERENCES

[1] Siegel RL, Miller KD, Jemal A: Cancer statistics, 2018. *CA Cancer J Clin* 2018; 68(1): 7–30.

[2] Lehmann BD, Bauer JA, Chen X, et al. Identification of human triple-negative breast cancer subtypes and preclinical models for selection of targeted therapies. *J Clin Invest* 2011;121:2750-2767.

[3] Arce-Salinas C, Riesco-Martinez MC, Hanna W, et al. Complete response of metastatic androgen receptor-positive breast cancer to biclutamide: Case report and review of the literature. *J Clin Oncol* 2014;34:e21-e24.

[4] Kast K, Link T, Friedrich K, et al. Impact of breast cancer subtypes and patterns of metastasis on outcome. *Breast Cancer Res Treat* 2015;150:621-629.

[5] Atchley DP, Albarracin CT, Lopez A, et al. Clinical and pathologic characteristics of patients with BRCA-positive and BRCA-negative breast cancer. *J Clin Oncol* 2008;26:4282-4288.

[6] Karami F, Mehdipour P. A comprehensive focus on global spectrum of BRCA1 and BRCA2 mutations in breast cancer. *Biomed Res. Int* 2013;2013:928562.

[7] Mavaddat N, Barrowdale D, Andrulis IL, et al. Pathology of breast and ovarian cancers among BRCA1 and BRCA2 mutation carriers: results from the Consortium of Investigators of Modifiers of BRCA1/2 (CIMBA). *Cancer Epidemiol Biomarkers Prev* 2012;21:134-147.

[8] Kratz J, Burkard M, O'Meara T, et al.: Incorporating Genomics Into the Care of Patients With Advanced Breast Cancer. *Am Soc Clin Oncol Educ Book* 2018; 38:56–64.

[9] Feng Y, Spezia M, Huang S, et al. Breast cancer development and progression: Risk factors, cancer stem cells, signaling pathways, genomics, and molecular pathogenesis. *Genes Dis* 2018; 5(2): 77–106.

[10] Lehmann BD, Pietenpol JA, Tan AR: Triple-negative breast cancer: molecular subtypes and new targets for therapy. *Am Soc Clin Oncol Educ Book* 2015;e31–9.

[11] Lee A, Djamgoz MBA: Triple negative breast cancer: Emerging therapeutic modalities and novel combination therapies. *Cancer Treat Rev.* 2018; 62:110–22.

[12] Tung NM, Garber JE. BRCA1/2 testing: therapeutic implications for breast cancer management. *Br J Cancer* 2018; 119(2): 141–52.

[13] Tutt A, Tovey H, Cheang MCU, et al. Carboplatin in BRCA1/2-mutated and triple-negative breast cancer BRCAness subgroups: the TNT Trial. *Nat Med* 2018; 24(5): 628–37. doi: 10.1038/s41591-018-0009-7.

[14] Robson M, Im SA, Senkus E, et al. Olaparib for Metastatic Breast Cancer in Patients with a Germline BRCA Mutation. *N Engl J Med.* 2017; 377(6): 523–33.

[15] Robson ME, Tung N, Conte P, Im SA, Senkus E, Xu B, et al. OlympiAD final overall survival and tolerability results: Olaparib versus chemotherapy treatment of physician's choice in patients with a germline BRCA mutation and HER2-negative metastatic breast cancer. *Ann Oncol* 2019;30(4):558-566. doi: 10.1093/annonc/mdz012.

[16] Litton JK, Rugo HS, Ettl J, Hurvitz SA, Gonçalves A, Lee K-H, et al. Talazoparib in Patients with Advanced Breast Cancer and a Germline BRCA Mutation. *N. Engl. J. Med* 2018;379:753–763. doi: 10.1056/NEJMoa1802905.

[17] Schmid P, Adams S, Rugo HS, Schneeweiss A, Barrios CH, Iwata H, et al. Atezolizumab and nab-paclitaxel in advanced triple-negative breast cancer. *N Engl J Med* 2018;379(22):2108-21. https://doi.org/10.1056/NEJMoa1809615.

[18] Kok M, Voorwerk L, Horlings H, et al. Adaptive phase II randomized trial of nivolumab after induction treatment in triple negative breast cancer (TONIC trial): Final response data stage I and first translational data. doi: 10.1200/JCO.2018.36.15_suppl.1012 *Journal of Clinical Oncology* 36, no.15_suppl (May 20 2018) 1012-1012.

[19] ClinicalTrials.gov. Study of single agent pembrolizumab (MK-3475) versus single agent chemotherapy for metastatic triple negative breast cancer (MK-3475-119/KEYNOTE-119). https://clinicaltrials.gov/ct2/show/NCT02555657. Accessed May 15, 2019.

[20] Adams S, Loi S, Toppmeyer D, Cescon DW, De Laurentiis M, Nanda R, et al. Pembrolizumab monotherapy for previously untreated, PD-L1-positive, metastatic triple-negative breast cancer: cohort B of the phase II KEYNOTE-086 study. *Ann Oncol* 2019;30(3):405-411. doi: 10.1093/annonc/mdy518.

[21] Rampurwala M, Wisinski KB, O'Regan R. Role of the androgen receptor in triple-negative breast cancer. *Clin Adv Hematol Oncol* 2016;14:186-193.

[22] Gerratana L, Basile D, Buono G, et al. Androgen receptor in triple negative breast cancer: A potential target for the targetless subtype. *Cancer Treat Rev* 2018; 68: 102–10.

[23] Gucalp A, Tolaney S, Isakoff SJ, et al. Phase II trial of bicalutamide in patients with androgen receptor-positive, estrogen receptor-negative metastatic Breast Cancer. *Clin Cancer Res* 2013; 19(19): 5505–12.

[24] Bonnefoi H, Grellety T, Tredan O, et al. A phase II trial of abiraterone acetate plus prednisone in patients with triple-negative androgen receptor positive locally advanced or metastatic breast cancer (UCBG 12-1). *Ann Oncol* 2016;27(5): 812–8.

[25] Traina TA, Miller K, Yardley DA, Eakle J, Schwartzberg LS, O'Shaughnessy J, et al. Enzalutamide for the Treatment of Androgen Receptor-Expressing Triple-Negative Breast Cancer. *J Clin Oncol* 2018;36(9):884-890. doi: 10.1200/JCO.2016.71.3495.

[26] ClinicalTrials.gov. Efficacy and safety study of enzalutamide in combination with paclitaxel chemotherapy or as monotherapy versus placebo with paclitaxel in patients with advanced, diagnostic-positive, triple-negative breast cancer (ENDEAR). https://clinicaltrials.gov/ct2/show/NCT02929576. Accessed May 15, 2019.

[27] Cardoso F, Senkus E, Costa A, et al.: *4th ESO-ESMO International Consensus Guidelines for Advanced Breast Cancer* (ABC 4). *Ann Oncol* 2018; 29(8):1634–57.

[28] Dent R, Trudeau M, Pritchard KI, et al. Triple-negative breast cancer: clinical features and patterns of recurrence. *Clin Cancer Res* 2007;13:4429-4434.

[29] Carey LA, Dees EC, Sawyer L, et al. The triple negative paradox: primary tumor chemosensitivity of breast cancer subtypes. *Clin Cancer Res* 2007;13:2329-2334.

[30] Petrucelli N, Daly MB, Pal T. BRCA1 and BRCA2-associated hereditary breast and ovarian cancer. GeneReviews®. Available at: https://www.ncbi.nlm.nih.gov/books/NBK1247. Accessed May 20, 2019.

[31] National Comprehensive Cancer Network. NCCN Clinical Practice Guidelines in Oncology. Genetic/familial high-risk assessment: breast and ovarian. https://www.nccn.org/professionals/physician_gls/PDF/genetics_screening.pdf. Accessed May 20, 2019.

[32] El Hachem G, Gombos A, Awada A. Recent advances in understanding breast cancer and emerging therapies with a focus on luminal and triple-negative breast cancer. F1000Res 2019. pii: F1000 *Faculty Rev*-591. doi: 10.12688/f1000research.17542.1. eCollection 2019. https://doi.org/10.12688/f1000research.17542.1.

[33] Esteva FJ, Hubbard-Lucey VM, Tang J, Pusztai L. Immunotherapy and targeted therapy combinations in metastatic breast cancer. *Lancet Oncol* 2019;20(3):e175-86. https://doi.org/10.1016/S1470-2045(19)30026-9.

[34] Heimes AS, Schmidt M. Atezolizumab for the treatment of triple-negative breast cancer. *Expert Opin Investig Drugs* 2019;28(1):1-5. https://doi.org/10.1080/13543784.2019.1552255.

[35] Oualla K, El-Zawahry HM, Arun B, et al. Novel therapeutic strategies in the treatment of triple-negative breast cancer. *Ther Adv Med Oncol* 2017;9(7):493-511. doi: 10.1177/1758834017711380.

In: Understanding a Cancer Diagnosis
Editors: W. P. dos Santos et al.
ISBN: 978-1-53617-520-28
© 2020 Nova Science Publishers, Inc.

Chapter 2

MORPHOLOGICAL DECOMPOSITION TO DETECT AND CLASSIFY LESIONS IN MAMMOGRAMS

Sidney Marlon Lopes de Lima[1],
Abel Guilhermino da Silva Filho[1]
and Wellington Pinheiro dos Santos[2],*

[1]Center of Informatics, Federal University of Pernambuco,
Recife, Brazil
[2]Department of Biomedical Engineering,
Federal University of Pernambuco, Recife, Brazil

ABSTRACT

According to the World Health Organization, breast cancer is the main cause of cancer death among adult women in the world. It is noteworthy, however, that this disease may have mortality rates much higher than official statistics. That is because in developing and underdeveloped countries, negligence still affects the determination of the pathological

---

* Corresponding Author's Email: wellington.santos@ufpe.br.

causes that lead to death. From the clinical point of view, mammography is still the most effective diagnostic technology, given the wide diffusion of the use and interpretation of the images. According to the state-of-the-art lesions classification on mammograms, wavelets have produced the best results from the viewpoint of performance, whereas in the pre-processing phase, they decompose the original image into detailed images (vertical, horizontal, and diagonal), and approximation images in order to have the shape and texture attributes extracted from these component images. We propose a class of Morphological Decomposition inspired by wavelets in order to decomposition in regions of interest on mammograms. The method employs non-linear low-pass and high-pass filters based on Mathematical Morphology. We used 355 images of fatty breast tissue of IRMA database, with 233 normal instances (no lesion), 66 benign cases and 56 malignant cases. Classification was performed by using SVM and ELM networks with modified kernels, in order to optimize accuracy rates, reaching 96.56%. Considering the ratio between accuracy and training time, our proposal proved to be 20 times superior to the best case of the state-of-the-art.

Keywords: breast cancer, mammography, morphological decomposition, wavelets, mathematical morphology

INTRODUCTION

Changes in the urban population lifestyle and in industrialized countries have increased the percentage of obese female adults. As breast cancer is directly influenced by obesity, sedentary lifestyle accompanied by poor eating habits can influence the increased incidence of the disease [1]. Thus, the expectation is that breast cancer remains to be the leading cause of cancer death among adult women in the world [1].

In 2003, obesity affected 33.2% of adult women in the United States [2]. In 2012, the percentage of obese women was 36.1% [3]. By considering the ethnic group composed only by black adult women, obesity affects nearly 60% of them [3].

In Western Europe, obesity rates grow, but not as fast as in the United States [4, 5]. In the UK, for example, obesity afflicted 23% of women in 2003. In 2012, the percentage of obese women was 25.1% [6]. In the developing countries of Latin America, such as Brazil and Mexico, the process of industrialization is recent compared to the same process in the US and in the UK. Obesity, however, is quite high. In Mexico, in 2000, obesity affected 28.6% of women [6]. In 2012, 37.5% of Mexican women were obese [6].

As obesity directly influences breast cancer [7], there is a high incidence of breast lesions in industrialized countries. In Western Europe, for example, breast cancer incidence reached more than 90 new cases for each group of 100,000 women per year [8]. While in East Africa, an area economically based on agricultural and handicraft, the incidence is of 30 new cases per 100,000 women [8]. Despite the high incidence of breast cancer in Western Europe, mortality rates are relatively low; one female patient dies in each group of six women patients, while in East Africa one woman dies for each two sick women [8]. One of the causes is that patients from East Africa do not have easy access to image diagnosis. Therefore, breast cancer is usually detected in advanced stages. Additionally, this fact may lead to the need of mastectomies, mutilating surgeries in which the suspicious mammary tissue is completely removed [9].

The loss of breast tissue causes, in general, a serious damage to the woman's self-esteem: this may lead her to a state of chronic depression. The reason is that mastectomy affects the woman's perception of her own sexuality and image as a person. Then, in order to reduce deaths and radical surgeries, such as mastectomy, early detection is required. In this sense, self-examination by touch is not sufficient: the availability of imaging diagnosis technologies is fundamental once, in some cases, tumours take about ten years to become palpable [9].

In undeveloped regions, death rates due to breast cancer are extremely high; however, the incidence rates in these regions should remain stable. The reason is that these areas still do not have the minimum conditions for an industrialization process; therefore, a significant portion of the population does not have sedentary habits that would influence the growth of the breast cancer rates. In these areas, obesity rates are not in a high degree of rise [10].

Influenced by the obesity increase in the adult female population, the incidence rates of breast cancer have been raising in the developed and in the developing countries lately. The difference is that, in developed countries, the mortality percentage is stabled or reduced [6, 7], as seen in Figure 1. While in developing regions, such as Brazil and Mexico, death percentage grows as there is a raise in breast cancer incidence [6, 7]. Thus, in developing countries, there is the junction of two adverse characteristics that directly influence breast cancer: obesity, as in developed regions, besides the difficulty to detect early lesions, as in undeveloped countries. Then, if measures are not taken, the expectation is that the mortality rates in developing regions exceed those of developed countries.

It is noteworthy that, both in developing and in undeveloped countries, breast cancer mortality rates may be much higher than those of official statistics. This occurs because these nations have difficulties in order to determine the pathological causes that led to death. Most deaths from natural causes that occur outside hospitals are not examined rigorously and they are classified in a generic way, for example; died of "old age," and "fever" [11]. In these countries, the number of deaths due to ill-defined natural causes and the lack of health care system assistance are in high proportion [11]. Then, official statistics in relation to deaths caused by breast cancer can be distorted.

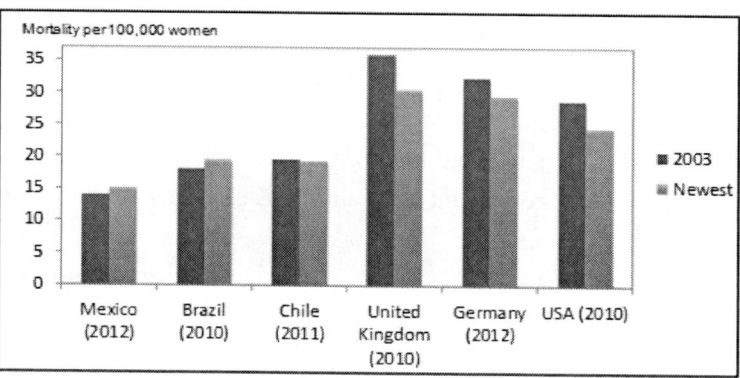

Source: [6].

Figure 1. Female mortality due to breast cancer (in the subtitle, each studied country is accompanied by the most recent year of data collection).

Following the pathway taken by developed countries and consequently reducing deaths caused by breast cancer is not trivial to developing countries. One of the measures would be the reduction of the percentage of obese female adults. Therefore, it is necessary to reduce pockets of poverty in the suburbs of large cities, because, in these areas, obesity is associated with poverty [12, 13].

In developing countries, such as Brazil and Mexico, pockets of poverty are formed in the outskirts of urban centers. This occurs because there is a tendency of the population to acquire an urban base; however, the migration process of the rural population towards urban centers occurs in a disorganized way. The cities do not offer jobs and dwelling houses compatible with the demand. Then, urban invasions are created. In these areas, there are poor living conditions and mobility, few recreational areas, low education levels, and little money in order to buy food that make up a healthy diet [12]. The countryside, however, cannot absorb the slum population. The land concentration in form of large latifundia is growing considerably [14]. Besides, a significant portion of these lands is unproductive, creating no job opportunities. In Brazil, paradoxically, more than 70% of the areas occupied by latifundia are unproductive [14]. Thus, in developing countries, pockets of poverty are one of the causes of obesity [12], although in some nations, such as Brazil, obesity is more common and has been spreading with greater intensity among richer classes [15, 16].

The other measure to reduce deaths caused by breast cancer in developing countries would be to universalize breast imaging exam [7]. Therefore, a better distribution of income is necessary so that poor adult women would pay for their own exams, or those countries would need an efficient public health system.

We discussed some of the major problems in developing countries in order to find ways to reduce deaths caused by breast cancer. The land concentration in unproductive latifundia, the ill income distribution and the inefficient public health services are recurrent problems in developing countries [17, 18, 19, 20, 21]. Thus, even with distorted and incomplete official data, death rates due to breast cancer in developing countries are expected to exceed those of developed countries in coming years.

Even for women with easy access to the breast imaging exam, the experience of a professional radiologist assumes a crucial role in finding and interpreting clinical data and developing an accurate diagnosis. A definite diagnosis is a particularly complex task due to the wide variability of cases, where many do not accurately fit in classical models and descriptions [22, 52]. Therefore, computational tools, named "second opinion," have been proposed in order to help the professional experts in diagnostic decisions.

The task of detecting and classifying mammary lesions using mammograms is highly dependent on the feature extraction stage, in which the regions of interest, clinically determined by using specialist knowledge, are pre-processed, and moments, statistics, and other measures are extracted. In breast cancer applications, the use of texture descriptors combined with segmentation methods is very common [24, 25, 26, 27, 28, 29, 30, 53, 54, 55, 57]. They aim to segregate the lesion from other image elements.

Several of these computational tools that employ segmentation techniques require specialist intervention during use phase [25, 26, 27, 28, 29, 30, 60]. Some types of human interventions, however, may require a large effort as a completely manual segmentation or as in fixing results of image processing techniques. The complexity is because a mammography usually has different degrees of intensity of gray levels. Then, only one threshold is rarely able to segment the entire edge of the mass. Removing or adding segmentations pieces freehand may compromise the feature extraction stage. The reason is that freehand work is likely to create a pattern that does not fit in gradient from the studied mammography. Thus, it is necessary to determine local thresholds or changes in parameters of image processing techniques to each micro-region of lesion through auxiliary software. Therefore, the most difficult interpretation and implementation part of the process is made by a specialist and not by computational solution. Thus, upon the completion of the segmentation, the radiologist is able to fully interpret lesion characteristics without the support of a computational tool.

More complex pre-processing approaches, however, have been being used in order to reach higher classification rates by modifying the feature dimensionality. One of the most successful techniques is the series of wavelets: each image of the region of interest is decomposed by a series of details images with different resolutions and a reduced and simplified version of the original image [23]. Features are extracted from these image components. In breast cancer applications, the state-of-the-art suggests classical wavelets decomposition, proposed by Mallat, using linear convolution filters [31]. Recent studies have been inspired by wavelets [54, 57]. Filters, however, are built by morphological operations and, then they are not linear. Morphological Decomposition has been successfully applied in remote sensing area [32, 33].

We propose a method of mammographies systematization inspired by wavelets of Mallat in image feature extraction, and ELM (Extreme Learning Machines) and SVM (Support Vector Machines) in classification. Our method reduces the decomposition into combined applications of high-pass and low-pass no linear filters; here, we use morphological operations in order to implement these filters. The feature extraction is made on images obtained from components of Morphological Decomposition using Zernike moments. The classification stage employs a multi-kernel approach, where different kernels are tested in ELM and SVM networks in order to maximize correct classification rate and minimize elements associated with misclassification [56, 58, 59].

For the experiments, we used the classification criteria for mammographic images defined according to the American College of Radiology, described on BI-RADS (Breast Imaging Reporting and Data) [34]. The goal of BI-RADS is to group the cases into three classes: normal (i.e., without cancer), benign lesion, and malignant lesion. We used 355 images of fatty breast tissue of IRMA database [35], with 233 normal instances, 66 benign cases, and 56 malignant cases. We generated synthetic instances of benign and malignant cases using linear combinations with random weights in order to balance our database, getting a final amount of 699 instances, with 233 instances for each class. The classification was performed by using SVM and ELM networks with modified kernels in order to optimize accuracy rates, reaching 96.56%. Considering the ratio between accuracy and training time, our proposal proved to be 20 times superior to state-of-the-art approaches.

This chapter is organized as follows: first, we present some of the most important related works; then, we present some of the fundamentals we used to build our method; followed by a presentation of the proposed method; after that, we show the experimental results and some discussion. Finally, we make general conclusions and discuss perspectives of our study.

RELATED WORKS

Several works have been being developed to solve the problem of the detection and classification of mammary lesions using mammograms, focusing on the feature extraction. Table 1 presents a list of some important works of the state-of-the-art, organized taking into account the ability to detect and classify lesions, the necessity of human intervention, a brief description of the feature extraction, and the amount of databases used in the experiments.

The works listed on Table 1 utilize different mammography databases. Selecting which database should be used is essential to get meaningful results, once getting satisfactory results using a determined database does not necessarily mean success when using another one. In this work, we used IRMA (Image Retrieval in Medical Applications) [34], a mammography database composed by two public databases: MiniMIAS (Mammographic Image Analysis Society database) [36] and DDSM (Digital Database for Screening Mammography) [37], and private mammograms. Therefore, this avoids methodological questions on the achieved accuracy rates, in relation to the set of used images.

Table 1 illustrates which methods of the state-of-the-art are designed to perform detection, and which ones are designed to perform classification. Detection means the ability to differentiate between normal tissue and lesion. Classification means the capacity to differentiate between benign and malignant lesions.

Table 1. Summary of main techniques for breast mass detection and/or classification

Authors	Description	Database Amount	Detection	Classification	Large human Intervention
Proposed model	Morphological Decomposition	1*	Yes	Yes	No
Nascimento et al. (2013) [23]	Conventional Wavelets	1	Yes	Yes	No
Pereira et al. (2014) [30]	Genetic algorithm	1	Yes	No	Yes
Wang et al. (2014) [29]	Region growing	1	Yes	No	Yes
Rouhi et al. (2014) [24]	CNN segmentation	2	No	Yes	Yes
Liu et al. (2014) [28]	Active contours	1	No	Yes	Yes
Tahmasbi et al. (2011) [25]	Zernike moments	1	No	Yes	Yes
Saki et al. (2013) [26]	Spiculation index	1	No	Yes	Yes
Tahmasbi et al. (2012) [27]	Cognitive Resonance	1	No	Yes	Yes

Table 1 shows the need of human intervention during training (learning phase) and/or using phases. Pereira et al. (2014) [30] aim to detect the presence of cancer. Image feature extraction consists of using a genetic algorithm in order to determine the amount of thresholds necessary for mass segmentation. The chromosomes of genetic algorithm are guided by the information in the image histogram. The paper reports that inadequate segmentations can be generated, thus, the radiologist intervenes in an indirect way. The professional manually segments the mammography in a mediolateral view, while the computational technique works in the corresponding craniocaudal view. Then, only regions of intersection between the work of the radiologist and the computational technique are considered. Besides lesions detection, Pereira et al. (2014) [30] also investigate the quality of the segmentations after indirect correction, performed by the radiologist. The work of Pereira et al. (2014) [30] does not report if the specialist intervention occurs only in training or also in use phase. The deduction is that it is necessary in both phases, since there is no change in description of the genetic algorithm parameters according to the indirect correction performed by the radiologist.

Wang et al. (2014) [29], similarly to Pereira et al. (2014), aim to detect the presence of mass. Image feature extraction requires human intervention in order to determine *the seed* based *region growing method*. Such approach seeks similarities among the neighboring pixels of the seed. The connections between neighboring pixels of the seed is also analyzed. Then, the initial grouping is expanded until no more pixels have to be added. When a seed is marked, the region growing method will achieve any type of segmentation, even in an image without lesion. Then, a series of geometric metrics, such as degree of circularity, is employed in order to study the mass shape in potential. The differentiation, concerning the presence or absence of cancer, uses these geometric variables as attributes. There is no specification if the marking of the seeds is performed by a radiologist or by the authors themselves. The intention, however, is that the computational solution be used by health specialists. Obviously, a maladjusted seed generates inadequate results and, thus, the lesion detection is damaged. In addition, health professionals may have difficulties with handling a computational tool to extract features from medical images, since the marking of the seeds is necessary both in training and in use phase.

Rouhi et al. (2014) [24] propose a classification of malignant and benign lesions. Thus, normal cases (no mass) are disregarded. Rouhi et al. (2014) [24] show two methodologies in order to analyse image feature extraction. The first one is based on region growing. The seed is obtained by a supervised neural network. The network is trained from manually selected seeds. There is no specification if the marking of the seeds is performed by a radiologist or by the authors themselves. The second methodology, with better precision, employs as image feature extraction the CNN technique (Cellular Neural Network). It has a similar paradigm to neural networks; however, synapse (communication) occurs only between neighboring neurons (cells). The CNN parameters are adjusted by a genetic algorithm whose objective function is to perform the intersection between manual segmentation done by the radiologist and the CNN technique production.

These two methodologies, proposed by Rouhi et al. (2014) [24], after training, are able to segment the lesion, and, thus, classify it between malignant and benign masses without the radiologist intervention.

Liu et al. (2014) [23] classify between malignant and benign lesions. This work uses the active contours technique as a method for mass segmentation. This paper reports imperfections in active contours results. These imperfections are manually excluded by the researchers. Then, geometric and texture metrics are used in the segmentation study, manually refined. The classification between malignant and benign lesions uses these metrics as input attributes. Manual refinement in segmentation is also required in use phase; otherwise, inadequate results can be generated. Liu et al. (2014) [28] also evaluate partially manual segmentation, refined by the authors. It is compared to the completely manual one, performed by a radiologist.

Tahmasbi et al. (2011) [25] employ a methodology with Zernike moments as the main image feature extraction. They are used in order to describe both shape and mass neighborhood region. Regarding the lesion shape, Zernike moments are projected in the segmentation done manually by the radiologist. The classification between malignant and benign lesions uses as the parameter the results of these projections.

Saki et al. (2013) [26] extend the work of their team, approved in Tahmasbi et al. (2011). Thus, normal cases (no mass) are disregarded. Image feature extraction employs some of Zernike moments and also includes a series of statistical variables, such as contrast and average grayscale of lesion and its neighborhood. In the work of Saki et al. (2013) [26], the mass is manually segmented by the radiologist. The spiculation index is also calculated. Spicules are radiating lines that start from the center towards the edge and the neighboring regions of the mass.

Tahmasbi et al. (2012) [27] extend the works to the concept of cognitive resonance. Then, characteristics approved in Saki et al. (2013) are mapped to a set of linguistic dialects inspired by radiological terms. Thus, a context-free grammar is developed. The classification between malignant and benign lesions uses this grammar as an input attribute.

Liu et al. (2014) [28], Tahmasbi et al. (2011) [25], Saki et al. (2013) [26], and Tahmasbi et al. (2012) [27] are not feasible to clinical practice as segmentation and/or refinements are necessary during use phase of computational solution. Radiologists have a demand of patients, thus, a lengthy process such as manual segmentation is not possible as part of their regular duty. In addition, the radiologist, when segmenting a lesion, is fully capable of interpreting the lesion characteristics without the support of a computational tool. Furthermore, human intervention can make the process lengthy, stressful and more error-prone. In addition, health professionals may have difficulties with handling a computational tool to extract features from medical images.

The works that require specialist intervention do not deal with the original image. The mass of interest is detected and segmented from other mammography information directly from the radiologist. Once these images, handled by specialists, are not disclosed, the replica of this type of project becomes impractical. Their achieved results are not totally comparable to others, due to the use of distinct metrics. Therefore, applications highly dependent on human intervention are not easily reproducible.

Nascimento et al. (2013) [23] propose a method in order to detect and classify masses based on wavelets decomposition. As such approach avoids the need of a specialist intervention, we adopted it and replicated it herein in order to improve this approach. In addition, other works of the state-of-the-art reviewed here do not have mechanisms in order to detect and classify lesions in a hybrid way. They are allocated to one aim or the other, while both Nascimento et al. (2013) [23] and we have methodologies in order to detect and classify masses. Thus, there are no unfair comparisons. The proposed methodology obtained an advantage about 20 times superior, taking into account the ratio between classification accuracy and computational cost, when compared to the best result of the state-of-the-art.

Nascimento et al. (2013) compared three types of families based on wavelets: Bi-orthogonal 3.7, Daubechies-8, and Symlet 8 [23]. The decomposition of the 128x128 mammogram is performed at two levels. Then, the images from the first and second levels are adjusted to the dimensions 64x64 and 32x32, respectively. The strategy adopted by Nascimento et al. (2013) is to smooth the image components by calculating the local energies normalized by the total image energy. Afterwards, the SVD (Singular Value Decomposition) technique is applied over all the smoothed images in order to reduce the amount of data necessary to form the feature vectors and, consequently, reducing the dimensionality of the classification problem.

BACKGROUND

Breast and Mass Classification

IRMA database description details the breast region description, as can be seen in Figure 2. In young women breasts, there is usually low adipose (fat) tissue: the breasts are dense. Muscles and others breast tissues (parenchyma) occupy most part of the breast.

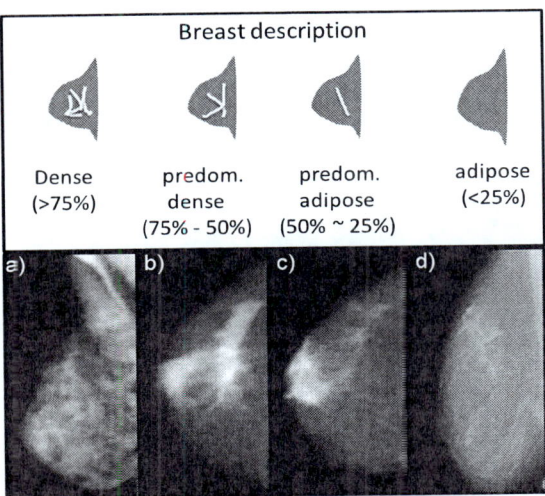

Source: [34].

Figure 2. Breast classification and description.

In a dense breast, parenchyma occupies more than 75% of breast tissue. In a predominantly dense breast, parenchyma occupies between 50% and 75% of breast tissue, whilst, in a predominantly adipose breast, parenchyma occupies between 25% and 50% of breast tissue. In an adipose breast, there is low parenchyma, less than 25% of breast tissue, and much more adipose tissue.

Adipose breasts are characteristic of elderly patients. There is a tendency of muscles and other parenchyma tissues being replaced by adipose tissue.

IRMA database description also provides mass classification information according to BI-RADS criteria. Masses are classified into five groups: regular, lobular, microlobulated, irregular and spiculated, as can be seen in Figure 3. A regular mass has benign characteristics, while a spiculated lesion has very high chances of being malignant. A regular mass presents a smooth edge with few variations. A lobular lesion has a wavy contour. A microlobulated mass presents smalls waves in the edge. A spiculated lesion has radiant lines in its margins. Finally, an irregular mass has, obviously, an irregular shape. An irregular mass does not fit the description of any other group.

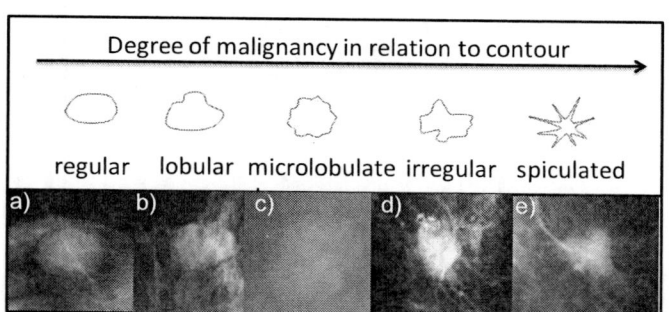

Source: The authors.

Figure 3. Classification of breast masses according to their contours.

In relation to density, Brazil's National Institute of Cancer (INCA) classifies masses into five groups: heterogeneous, fat, low density, isodense and high-density, as shown in Figure 4. A high-density mass presents a density higher than tissue density. Isodense masses have density equals to skin. Low-density masses have density lower than tissue density. Fat lesions have low-density and contain fats in their neighboring. Finally, heterogeneous masses have low-density and are partially occupied by mammary parenchyma.

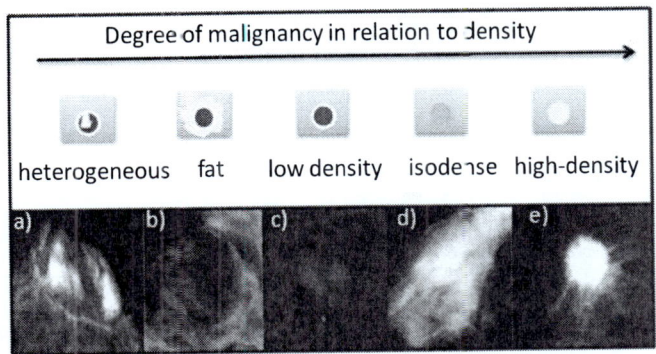

Source: The authors.

Figure 4. Classification of breast masses according to their densities.

Theoretically, malignant tumors have a higher density than tissue density, whilst benign masses have lower density. BI-RADS, for instance, mentions that fat lesions are massively benign [34].

Database

IRMA database is composed by some private mammography databases and two public databases, namely [35]:

- Mini-MIAS (Mammographic Image Analysis Society database) [36];
- DDSM (Digital Database for Screening Mammography) [37].

The database documentation details the scanning method of breast imaging, presenting the imaging directions. These directions can be mediolateral and cranio-caudal. IRMA documentation also specifies if it was imaged the right or the left breast. Lesions and breast tissues are also classified according to BI-RADS criteria, as mentioned before [34].

All available database cases were investigated. There are not heterogeneous, fat and low-density masses, explained in the previous sections. All lesions are isodense and high-density.

It is quite common the presence of undesirable artifacts in digital mammograms due to the lack of care at the digitalization or unexpected variations inherent to the acquisition process, e.g., calibration problems. These artifacts are usually present as random elements over the breast, like tapes, trowels, and handwritten and digital notes, as can be seen in the Mini-MIAS [36] and DDSM [37] databases. Furthermore, it is also common grooves and greases caused by fingerprints. These elements contribute to increase image analysis difficulties. IRMA database avoids these situations by furnishing the regions of interest (ROI) clinically selected using specialist knowledge.

Image Analyses Domain

A spiculated mass can be benign and a regular mass can be malign as well. These assessments can be achieved through a biopsy surgery and the patient medical history acquired by anamnesis process. Mammography is just one of the items in order to perform the adequate diagnosis and, therefore, choose the appropriate treatment for the patient. Consequently, it is not possible to determine a spiculated lesion as a benign mass, for example, just analyzing mammographic images. Therefore, All IRMA contradictory cases, i.e., benign spiculated masses and malignant circumscribed masses, were discarded. Once the necessary focus of clinical decision support systems is aiding health professionals to make accurate diagnosis, we did not dealt with cases depending on the clinical information of the patient or other information that could be easily obtained by the specialist using day-by-day clinical procedures.

Balancing Databases

IRMA also provides cases of calcification, architectural distortion, and asymmetry. We did not deal with these types of lesions. The area occupied by a calcification, for example, is very small in comparison with the breast area. Our proposal addresses only the adipose (fatty) breast tissues, because mammary parenchyma gray levels in dense breasts images are very close to mass regions gray levels. In dense breasts cases, usually of young patients, commonly it is not possible to identify the edge lesion, including for experienced radiologists.

Given the appropriate restriction, IRMA provides 355 cases of adipose (fatty) breasts. There are 233 normal cases (normal tissue, without lesions), 66 benign mass cases and 56 malignant lesion cases. In order to use IRMA database in classification applications, we balance this dataset, generating 167 and 177 synthetic benign and malignant instances, respectively. The proposed methodology is creating artificial instances based on real image features instances. Therefore, a vector of random weights is created, with the same amount of artificial class cases. The weights uniformly vary from 0 to 1. These weights are used to form linear combinations of the real instances, in order to calculate the synthetic instances.

Morphological Operations

Mathematical Morphology is a complete theory of nonlinear processing extensively used in digital image processing. It is based on shape transformations preserving the object relations of inclusion. Its fundamental operators are called *erosion* and *dilation* [38, 39, 40, 41]. Furthermore, Mathematical Morphology can be considered a constructive theory, because all operators are built using erosions and dilations as bases. It turns possible the construction of several operators designed to specific applications, as image filtering, feature extraction and [38, 39, 40, 41].

Mathematically, erosion and dilation are formalized in accordance with the expressions of Equations 1 and 2, respectively [38, 39, 40, 41].

$$\varepsilon_g(f)(u) = \bigcap_{v \in S} f(v) \vee \bar{g}(u-v), \tag{1}$$

$$\delta_g(f)(u) = \bigcup_{v \in S} f(v) \wedge g(u-v), \tag{2}$$

where $f: S \to [0,1]$ and $g: S \to [0,1]$ are normalized monospectral images with support $S \subseteq \mathbb{N}^2$, the operators $\cup$ and $\vee$ are associated with the maximum operator, whilst $\cap$ and $\wedge$ are associated with the minimum operator; $\bar{g}(u) = 1 - g(u)$ is the negation of $g(u)$, $\forall\, u \in S$; $g: S \to [0,1]$, is the structure element of the respective erosion and dilation [38, 39, 40, 41].

The erosion transforms the original image in such a way to make the negative of the structure element to incase in the original image, i.e., the original image $f(u)$ will be modified to make areas similar to $\bar{g}(u)$ increase, to incase $\bar{g}(u)$ [41]. If we associate the 1's to the absolute white and the 0's to the absolute black, we will perceive that the erosion results in the augment of the darkest areas and the elimination of the brightest areas [41].

The dilation transforms the original image in such a way to make the structure element to incase in the original image, i.e., the original image $f(u)$ will be modified to make areas similar to $g(u)$ increase, to incase $g(u)$ [41]. If we associate the 1's to the absolute white and the 0's to the absolute black, we will perceive that the dilation results in the augment of the brightest areas and the elimination of the darkest areas [41].

The implementation of a dilation of an image $f(u)$ followed by an erosion, with the same structure element $g(u)$, is known as *closing* $\phi_g(f)(u)$. *Closing* as its name suggests closes (approximate) spaces among objects in image. If we associate the 1's to mass shape and the 0's to breast tissue, we will perceive that *closing* fills failures in shape edge.

The application of an erosion followed by a dilation, also with the same structuring element is known as *opening* $\gamma_g(f)(u)$ [41]. *Opening* as its name suggests opens (depart) spaces among objects in image. If we associate the

1's to mass shape and the 0's to breast tissue, we will perceive that *opening* smoothes mass edge, eliminating nozzles at shape contour.

Morphological Spectrum

Let us consider a normalized monospectral image $f: S \to [0,1]$. The residual area resulting from the k-th opening operation, where $k \geq 0$, by the structure element $g: S \to [0,1]$, is given by the expression on Equation 3 as following [41].

$$V(k) = \sum_{u \in S} \gamma_g^k(f)(u). \tag{3}$$

The mathematical expression in Equation 4 describes in details the discrete accumulated density function, $\Xi: Z_+ \to [0,1]$ associated to image $f: S \to [0,1]$ [41].

$$\Xi[k] = 1 - \frac{V(k)}{V(0)}. \tag{4}$$

The discrete density function, also known as the pattern spectrum or morphological spectrum, is presented on Equation 5 [41]. The pattern or morphological spectrum can be used as a very precise feature extractor based on shape, because the morphological theory guarantees that each binary image has unique representation based on this spectrum [41]. The pattern spectrum can be employed in pattern recognition applications as a type of digital signature [41].

$$\xi[k] = \Xi[k+1] - \Xi[k]. \tag{5}$$

In order to calculate the morphological spectrum, we have to perform the operations until the algorithm converges, i.e., when we get a null image, which returns null residual area ($V(k) = 0$). Different mammograms require k-different iterations in order to conclude the morphological spectrum. Therefore, trying to avoid the problem of different-sized morphological spectra, we represented these spectra by using seven statistics, namely: mean, standard deviation, mode, median, kurtosis, minimum, and maximum value.

Let us consider a sphere of radius R, with a structure element in a disc shape. The correspondent morphological spectrum will be an impulse. By changing the radius size to 2R, the spectrum will remain to be an impulse. This fact illustrates the singular characteristic of morphological spectra as unique shape identifiers. Therefore, irregularities in mammary mass edges results in low amplitude variations in morphological spectra.

Morphological spectra may be useful in mammography study, because they present as advantage the ability to disregard low amplitude variations in mass edges. Furthermore, pattern spectra can be used as unique representations of tumor shape, regardless of size.

Image Representation Using Wavelets

A wavelet $\psi(t)$ is a wave-like function which obeys to the following conditions:

$$\int_{-\infty}^{+\infty} \psi(t) dt = 0, \tag{6}$$

$$\int_{-\infty}^{+\infty} |\psi(t)|^2 dt < +\infty. \tag{7}$$

The wavelet $\psi(t)$ is called a mother wavelet, with child wavelets $\psi_{a,b}(t)$ translated and scaled versions of the mother wavelet, given by:

$$\psi_{a,b}(t) = \frac{1}{\sqrt{a}} \psi\left(\frac{t-b}{a}\right), \tag{8}$$

where a and b are the scaling and the translating factors, respectively. Given a continuous time signal $x(t)$, its continuous wavelet transform, $X(a,b)$, is given by:

$$X(a,b) = \int_{-\infty}^{+\infty} x(t) \psi_{a,b}^{*}(t) dt, \tag{9}$$

where * means the conjugate.

The wavelet transform applied to the image processing can be implemented in a two-dimensional way. Mallat proposed a discrete wavelet transform of a unidimensional signal through the decomposition a series of signal components generated by discrete high-pass and low-pass filters [31].

Wavelets decomposition, proposed by Mallat, are very in order to represent images using a multi-resolution representation. Then, the original image is decomposed into images with different resolutions. Figure 5 shows the two-dimensional wavelet decomposition algorithm considering just one level of resolution. The image A_j is convoluted by $h(n)$ and $g(n)$ filters. The two images, resulting from the convolution, are decimated by a factor of 2, where odd lines and columns are excluded. Afterwards, in the end of each level, Mallat's algorithm generates an approximation image, obtained by low pass filtering, and three detail images, resulting from high pass oriented filtering.

An approximation image (LL) consists of a representation of the original image without details, resulting from the application of a low pass filter. It appears to be a blurred version of the original image, due to the reduction of the number of gray levels.

A detail image aims to represent the original image in high frequency. A high pass filter enhances the elements present in the edge of the original image. At each level of wavelets, Mallat's algorithm generates three detail images: one to horizontal details (HL), another to vertical details (LH), and finally, to diagonal details (HH). The next level decomposition process uses, as source, the approximation image from the level immediately preceding.

Figure 6 presents the wavelets decomposition process into levels, using Daubechies 8. The goal of this technique is to decompose the original image in an approximation image and three detail images, at each level.

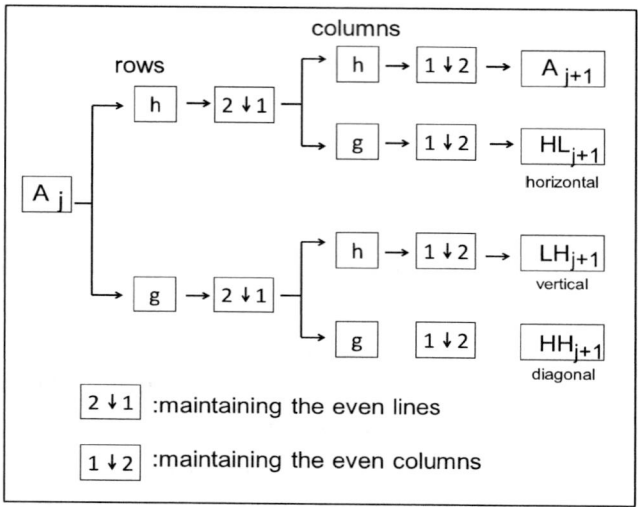

Source: The authors.

Figure 5. Wavelet decomposition algorithm for two-dimensional wavelets, considering just one resolution level.

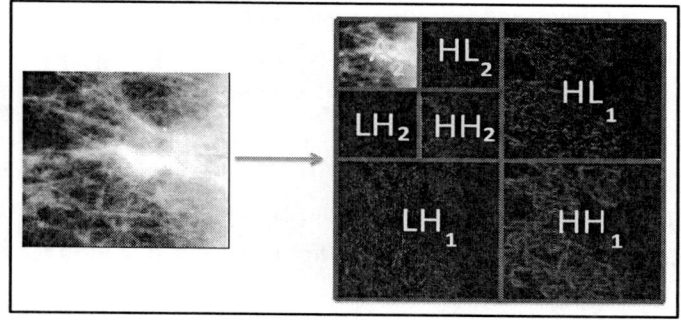

Source: The authors.

Figure 6. Illustration of wavelet decomposition in 2 levels, based on Daubechies 8 function.

Zernike Moments

The Zernike polynomials are a basis of complex orthogonal polynomials. The mathematical expression of the radial Zernike polynomials is the following, illustrated by Equation 10:

$$R_{n,m} = \sum_{s=0}^{(n-|m|)/2} (-1)^s \frac{(n-s)!}{s!(((n+|m|)/2)-s)!(((n-|m|)/2)-s)!} p^{n-2s},$$

(10)

where n is a non-negative integer representing the radial polynomial order; m is a non-zero integer, for $n - |m|$ non-negative and even; p is the distance between the center and a point of the polynomial function. The computation of Zernike basis function, expressed in polar coordinates, is formalized by Equation 11, as following:

$$V_{n,m}(p,\theta) = R_{n,m}(p)e^{jm\theta}, \lfloor p \rfloor \leq 1$$

(11)

where θ is the angle formed between the line segment that joins the center to point p and the axis coordinate, also named the azimuthal angle. The imaginary unit is given by $j = \sqrt{-1}$.

Since Zernike polynomials integrate an orthogonal basis, Zernike moments are able to represent image properties with no redundancy or overlap of information between the moments. Zernike moments are significantly dependent on scaling and translation. Nevertheless, their magnitudes are independent of the rotation angle of the object. Figure 7 illustrates the magnitude of the first Zernike moments in the unit disk.

Therefore, we can utilize them to describe shape characteristics of the objects of interest. Due to these qualities, Zernike moments have been used successfully to represent mammary regions of interest in mammograms [25, 26, 27, 51, 52]. Note that Zernike moment, with $n=0$, $m=0$, has an adequate shape in order to describe regular masses, while the moment with $n=5$, $m=5$, can describe spiculated mass which has lines from its center in direction to its margins, seen in Figure 3. Figure 8 shows an example of mass shape being descript by a Zernike moment, with $n=0$, $m=0$.

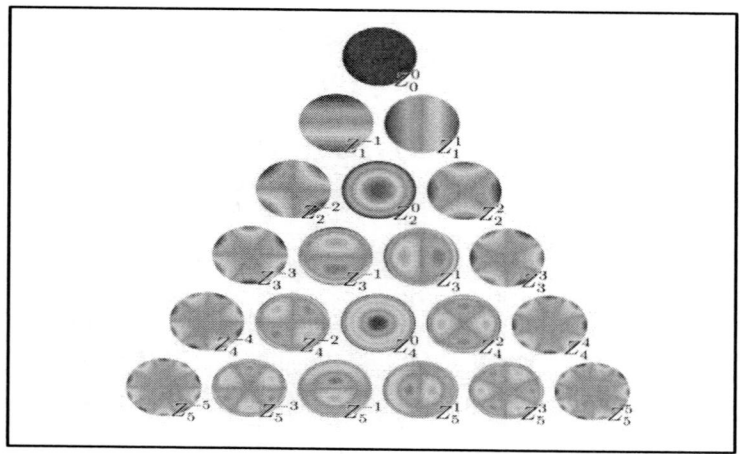

Source: [25].

Figure 7. Plots of the magnitude of Zernike basis functions in the unit disk.

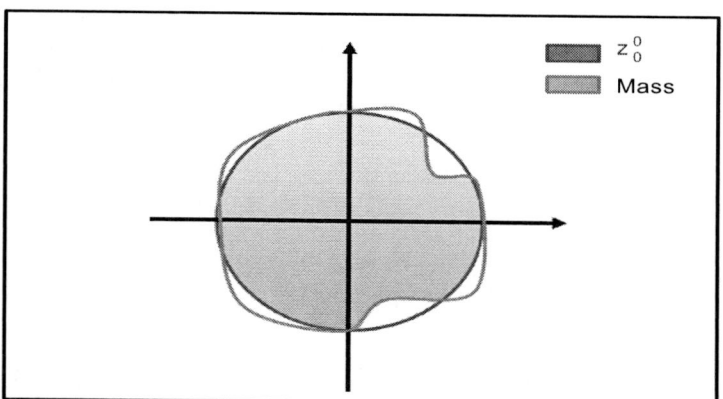

Source: The authors.

Figure 8. Description of mass shape and Zernike, $n=0$; $m=0$.

Extreme Learning Machines (ELM)

ELM networks have as the main characteristic high training speed and good data prediction abilities when compared to other networks used as classifiers. ELM networks have a single non-recursive hidden layer. They have as a remarkable characteristic the fast training process, composed by just a few steps. The weights of the hidden layer neurons are randomly determined, once their kernels are defined. The weights of the output neurons are determined by the calculation of the generalized pseudoinverse of Moore-Penrose [49]. This learning process is performed in batch mode, where all data is presented to the network before the calculation of the weights, in a single iteration. Once this learning algorithm is not based on gradient descent methods, ELM networks are not affected by local minima. Furthermore, it is not necessary to define neither a learning rate parameter nor a maximum of iterations, once this is a non-iterative algorithm.

Support Vector Machines (SVM)

SVM networks are single or multilayer networks with linear neurons in the output layer. These networks classify data by choosing the optimal hyperplanes in the output layer, which separate data within their respective classes, optimizing classification accuracy for the training set [50]. The best hyperplanes have the largest separation in relation to the given classes [50].

The original SVM training algorithm is able to deal with just two classes. Due to this limited binary nature, we used the LibSVM library, a computational library to classify data into multiple classes, once our problem of detection and classification of mammary lesions have three classes [50].

PROPOSED METHOD

Figure 9 shows the block diagram of the proposed design flow. First of all, mammographic images are preprocessed and have their histogram normalized, in order to associate the brightest pixels to absolute white and the darkest pixels to absolute black. Afterwards, images are decomposed by Morphological Decomposition.

Thereafter, they are extracted images feature vectors from the decomposed images. The classification phase use as input attributes these feature vectors in a concatenated way. Classification aims to group mammograms according to the American College of Radiology. Thus, cases are classified into three classes: normal (i.e., without mass), benign and malignant lesion.

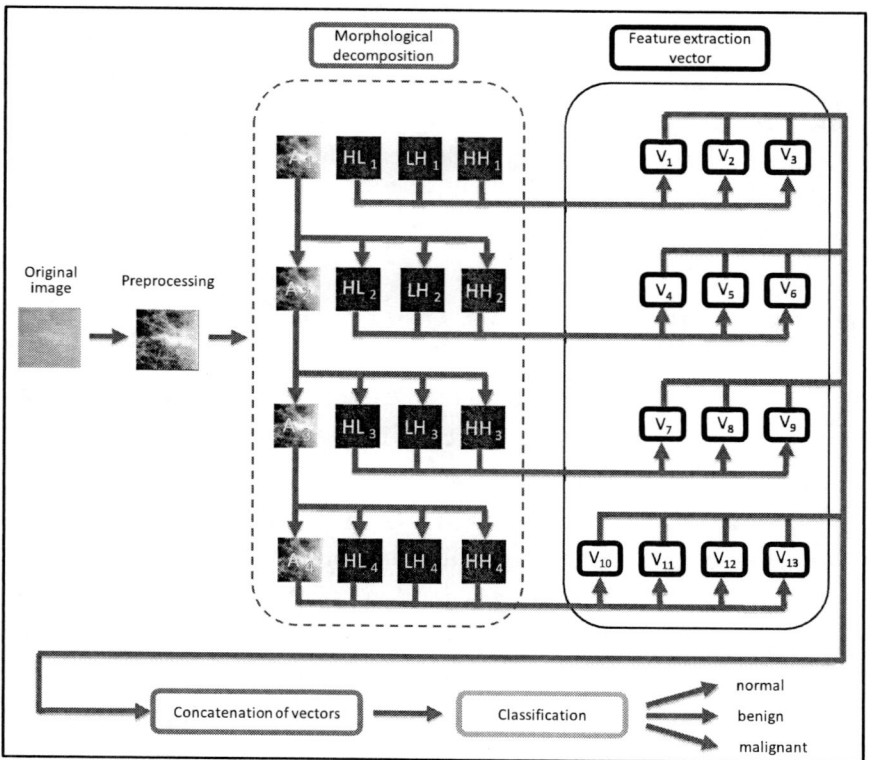

Source: The authors.

Figure 9. Block diagram of the proposed breast lesion detection and classification method.

Morphological Decomposition

In breast cancer applications, wavelets have produced notably results [23]. The classic wavelet proposed by Mallat causes decomposition in a series of images with different resolutions. Mallat decomposition uses linear convolution filters [31]. Recent studies have been inspired by wavelets in image processing area [32, 33]. Filters, however, are built by morphological operations and, then they are not linear.

In our decomposition, a class of Morphological Decomposition, inspired by wavelet, is created. Approximation image A is the result of the LPF (Low-Pass Filter) applied on original image, described in Equation (12):

$$LPF(f)(u) = \gamma_g^n \phi_g^n \gamma_g^n(f)(u), n = \text{level}, \forall u \in S \qquad (12)$$

The operation denoted by $\gamma_g^n(f)$ is named n-opening, where $n > 1$; $f: S \rightarrow K; g: S \rightarrow [0,1]$. Mathematically, $K = \{0, 1, \ldots 255\}$ where $K \in \mathbb{N}$. By following the formalization described in work of Santos et al. (2011), n-opening is proposed in Equation (13):

$$\gamma_g^n(f)(u) = \gamma_g \gamma_g \ldots \gamma_g(f)(u), \forall u \in S. \qquad (13)$$

Similarly, operation $\phi_g^n(f)$ is named n-closing, with $n > 1; f: S \rightarrow K; g: S \rightarrow [0,1]$, in Equation (14):

$$\phi_g^n(f)(u) = \phi_g \phi_g \ldots \phi_g(f)(u), \forall u \in S. \qquad (14)$$

The structuring element (g), relative to approximation image A, has dimension 3x3 and all its pixels are enabled.

In Equation (12), initially the n-opening eliminates nozzles in mass edge, with larger intensity as n increases. Thereafter, there is the merge with the n-closing which fills failures in lesion edge, with larger intensity as n increases. Imperfections in mass contour are quite common because there are different degrees of lighting and intensity in mammography images, due to image scanning process. Thus, the mass edge needs to be redone. Then, n-closing fills failures in lesion edge, this fact turns our methodology able in order to generate a uniform edge without a radiologist intervention as almost always occurs in state-of-the-art [25, 26, 27, 28, 29, 30]. At least, n-opening eliminating nozzles, yet remaining, in contour, the goal is to achieve an edge with uniform thickness.

In our class of Morphological Decomposition, the three detail images are derived from application of HPF (High-Pass Filter), described in Equation (15):

$$HPF(f)(u) = \delta_g^n(f)(u) - \varepsilon_g^n(f)(u), \text{n} = \text{level}, \forall\, u \in S. \qquad (15)$$

The operation formalized by $\delta_g^n(f)$ is called n-dilation, where $n > 1; S \to K; g: S \to [0,1]$. Its expression is in accordance with Equation (16):

$$\delta_g^n(f)(u) = \delta_g \delta_g \ldots \delta_g(f)(u), \forall\, u \in S. \qquad (16)$$

Similarly, the operation $\varepsilon_g^n(f)$ is n-erosion, with $n > 1; S \to K; g: S \to [0,1]$. n-erosion is formalized in Equation (17):

$$\varepsilon_g^n(f)(u) = \varepsilon_g \varepsilon_g \ldots \varepsilon_g(f)(u), \forall\, u \in S. \qquad (17)$$

The structuring elements (g), relative to detail images have dimension of 3x3. (g) of horizontal detail has only the center line enabled. (g) of vertical detail has only the center column enabled. At least, (g) of diagonal detail has the main and secondary diagonal enabled.

As number of levels n increases, the *n-dilation* operation successively expands the mass size. Conversely, as n increases, the *n-erosion* operation continuously reduces the mass dimension. Then, a subtraction between images resulting from the *n-dilation* and *n-erosion*, as formalized in Equation (15), is referents to mass edge detection. As n increases, the edge tends to have an increasingly thickness, since the difference between the *n-dilation* and *n-erosion* becomes larger.

As there is advance of levels, our Morphological Decomposition is able to process increasingly larger lesions. Regarding to mass dimension, as there are levels advance, the structure becomes able to only process lesions of large dimensions. The architecture, in levels, resembles successive operations on same original image, with structuring elements in ascending dimension. This fact occurs because the LPF application (properly the *n-opening*), described in Equation (12), causes a blurring in Approximation images A_{level}, with larger intensity as level decomposition increases. As there is advance of levels, Approximation images A_{level} lose resolution. Then, in first level, there is study of masses of all dimensions. While at higher levels, there is evaluation of large lesions. Herein this work we create a Morphological Decomposition architecture composed by four levels, from which we obtained 13 image components. We claim that this strategy is able to deal with several mass sizes.

The creation of our class of Morphological Decomposition as main technique of image feature extraction is not based on empiricism, or trial and error method. There was a deeper study of *American College of Radiology* rules. Furthermore, there was the image database analysis. Thus, it was found that the proposal of Morphological Decomposition is suitable in for detection and classification breast mass, compared to state-of-the-art.

Wavelets, proposed by Mallat [31], investigate image texture intensity, in multi-resolution. It is noteworthy that texture is essential in order to determine the lesion presence or absence, with several sizes. After mass detection, it is required classification between benign and malignant. In classical images and descriptions, Wavelets are enough in order to resolve this classification since, in radiological literature, there is an abrupt change in intensity (texture) of gray levels between benign and malignant lesions. While in images provided by IRMA database, this fact does not usually occur. All examined masses are isodense or high-density, thus their textures are very near. Then, in order to classify between benign and malignant lesions it is important to analyze mass shape. Thus, our class of Morphological Decomposition may be relevant. It maintains the characteristic of Wavelets which is the study of intensity of gray levels through the image decomposition, using a multi-resolution approach.

Furthermore, Morphological Decomposition has the advantage, over wavelets, the study of image morphology. In our class of Morphological Decomposition, the sequence of *n-opening* and *n-closing*, described in Equation (12), can redone the edge of the mass, vandalized in the image scanning process. Then, through our class of Morphological Decomposition, the proposed methodology is able to as detect as classify breast masses.

In our Morphological Decomposition, there are generated an approximation image and three detail images for each level, as shown in Figure 9. After decomposition, features are extracted from the detail images of all four levels. In addition, only approximation image of fourth and final level has its features described, respecting the theoretical foundation proposed by Mallat [31] and seen in Figure 6. In Mallat foundation, only the approximation image of last level composes the series of wavelets decomposition. The approximation images of previous levels only serve as input attribute for the level immediately posterior.

Feature Extraction Vector

Morphological Decomposition results in 13 images, as previously explained. Then, Zernike moments are applied in each one of these resulting images. Thus, there is extraction of 32 descriptors for each image, detailed in Table 2.

Table 2. The Zernike Moments studied

Zernike Moments		
Order(n)	Iteration (m)	Number of moments
3	1,3	
4	0,2,4	
5	1,3,5	
6	0,2,4,6	32
7	1,3,5,7	
8	0,2,4,6,8	
9	1,3,5,7,9	
10	0,2,4,6,8,10	

The descriptors by projection of Zernike moments are normalized between 0 and 1. In Table 2, the order n ranges from 3 to 10, in ascending order. The iteration module m should be less or equal to the given order n. All the differences $n = |m|$ must be multiple of 2.

Concatenation of Vectors

For each image from database, we use 416 descriptors. They relate to 32 Zernike moments extracted from 13 images decomposed by Morphological Decomposition. For all classifiers used in next phase, we use an input layer with 416 neurons, relating to image feature descriptors. All IRMA images have dimension 128x128.

Classification

The proposed breast cancer detection and classification methodology employs artificial neural networks as classifiers. We used the following network architectures: Extreme Learning Machines (ELM), and Support Vector Machines (SVM). ELM and SVM networks were adopted using a multi-kernel approach in order to discover the best configuration for the proposed feature extraction method, regarding classification performance, especially accuracy. These architectures were also chosen to allow comparisons with the state-of-the-art methods.

For all neural network architectures, we set 416 inputs, i.e., the dimensionality of the feature vectors: 416 features, with 32 Zernike moments for each of the 13 image components. For all neural networks we used, the number of neurons of the output layer equals the number of classes: three neurons, each one dedicated to identify one of the classes of interest established by BI-RADS criteria: normal (no lesion), benign, and malignant lesion.

Multi-Kernel Configurations

Considering artificial neurons as basic connective processing units, kernels are mathematical functions which define how the output is calculated from the inputs and their synaptic weights. Linear kernels, as those used in McCulloch-Pitts original artificial neurons, define the output as a linear combination between the weights vector and the input vector. These neurons are not able to solve nonlinearly separable problems, e.g., separating Gaussian-distributed data. However, Radial Basis Function (RBF) kernels deal with these problems adequately, once neural outputs are calculated by applying the Euclidian distance between inputs and weights to a Gaussian function.

Herein our proposal we suggest the variation of the nature of kernels in SVM and ELM networks, as an interesting strategy to maximize classification accuracy and minimize training time and computational cost.

Thus, for ELM we tested eight different types of kernels: RBF, linear, polynomial, wavelet transform, sigmoid, sine, hard limit, and tribas (triangular basis function) [49]. The proposed work has a methodological care on ELM configurations. We implemented cross-validation using the k-fold method with ten folds. Our objective was avoiding the influence of training and test set on results. The dataset was divided into ten subsets. In the first iteration, the first subset is used for testing, while the others are reserved to training. This continues until all subsets are used for testing. We defined ELM total accuracy as the simple mean of the accuracies obtained in each k-fold step. The ELM architecture has 100 neurons on hidden layer.

The strategy employed in SVM was the same as the one used with ELM networks, considering architecture, training and test stages. For SVM, we tested four different types of kernels: linear, polynomial, RBF, and sigmoid.

RESULTS

Table 3 shows the results of the ELMs neural networks in a multi-kernel approach. The best cases are emphasized in bold. The first and second criteria are the sample mean average and the standard deviation, respectively.

As a strategy for training and test we used the k-fold method with 10 folds. ELM networks achieved a maximum accuracy rate of 82.73% for linear kernels. Training time was considerably short. For RBF, linear, polynomial, and wavelet kernels, ELM classifiers could reach high percentage accuracy rate, with low dispersion of the results, independent of the data set arrangement.

Table 3. Results of feature extraction of proposed model by Morphological Decomposition. The classifiers are ELMs networks for grouping into 3 classes: normal, benign and malignant

	Train rate (%)	Test rate (%)	Train time (sec.)	Test time (sec.)
ELM, RBF	100.00 ± 0.00	82.15 ± 0.05	0.10 ± 0.04	0.01 ± 0.03
ELM, linear	99.92 ± 0.00	**82.73 ± 0.05**	0.05 ± 0.02	**0.00 ± 0.00**
ELM, polynomial	98.72 ± 0.01	80.71 ± 0.07	0.04 ± 0.03	0.01 ± 0.02
ELM, wavelet	100.00 ± 0.00	82.00 ± 0.05	0.12 ± 0.02	0.03 ± 0.04
ELM, sigmoid	34.78 ± 0.01	28.62 ± 0.05	0.03 ± 0.05	**0.00 ± 0.00**
ELM, sine	62.48 ± 0.02	45.21 ± 0.05	0.03 ± 0.03	**0.00 ± 0.00**
ELM, hard limit	34.10 ± 0.00	26.46 ± 0.04	0.04 ± 0.04	0.01 ± 0.02
ELM, tribas	33.33 ± 0.01	33.30 ± 0.06	**0.01 ± 0.02**	0.01 ± 0.02

Table 4. Results of feature extraction of proposed model by Morphological Decomposition. The classifiers are SVMs networks for grouping into 3 classes: normal, benign and malignant

	Train rate (%)	Test rate (%)	Train time (sec.)	Test time (sec.)
SVM, linear	**99.62 ± 0.00**	**96.56 ± 0.03**	0.63 ± 0.16	0.01 ± 0.01
SVM, polynomial	98.92 ± 0.00	93.92 ± 0.03	3.26 ± 3.79	0.01 ± 0.01
SVM, RBF	99.05 ± 0.00	79.43 ± 0.04	**0.25 ± 0.01**	0.03 ± 0.01
SVM, sigmoid	32.06 ± 0.02	28.04 ± 0.03	0.23 ± 0.01	0.01 ± 0.03

Table 4 displays the results obtained using SVM classifiers. Similarly to ELM classifiers, we also employed k-fold strategy. Taking into account accuracy rates, classifiers based on linear and polynomial kernels obtained superior performance to other classifiers. The configuration based on linear kernels achieved the best accuracy of all networks, getting 96.56% in distinction of normal, benign and malignant cases. Regarding the training time, SVM networks are not as fast as ELMs. By analyzing all metrics, SVM classifiers obtained stable low-dispersed results, except for just one case, using polynomial kernels, when the standard deviation of the training time was relatively high.

Herein this work we decided to replicate the proposal of Nascimento et al. (2013) [23] in order to perform comparisons between our proposal and such state-of-the-art method. Nascimento et al. (2013) uses three wavelets families: Biorthogonal 3.7, Daubechies 8, and Symlet 8 [23].

Another type of methodology was also employed. This time, the whole method was replicated. There is only one change, however. Morphological Decomposition is replaced by wavelets proposed by Mallat [31]. They are use families employed in work of Nascimento et al. (2013) [23]; Daubechies 8, Biorthogonal 3.7, and Symlet 8. The architecture contains four levels as well the methodology created for Morphological Decomposition. The reason for creation of this experiment is to investigate the relevance of our class of Morphological Decomposition in the proposed design flow.

We also investigated the performance of the morphological spectrum as part of the feature extraction process to describe breast lesions. We tested two 3x3 structure elements, square and cross, trying to investigate the effect of analysis given eight and four directions, respectively. Afterwards, seven statistics are measured from each pattern spectrum, in order to describe it, as previously explained in this chapter.

Table 5 shows results for all approaches compared with ours. SVM was the classifier. The reason is that SVM presented good results as proposed model as state-of-the-art [23]. We used three different types of kernels: linear, polynomial, and RBF.

Considering the configurations with linear kernel, our proposal reached an accuracy of 96.56%. With the approach proposed by Nascimento et al. (2013), a slightly less classification performance was reached, get an accuracy of 96.39%. However, except for the use of RBF kernels, training times spent using the approach of Nascimento et al. (2013) were considerably higher than times obtained with other approaches.

Table 5. Comparison between the proposed model and the state-of-the-art approaches

		Function	Train rate (%)	Test rate (%)	Train time (sec.)	Test time (sec.)
SVM, linear	Proposed model	--	99.62 ± 0.00	96.56 ± 0.03	0.63 ± 0.16	0.01 ± 0.01
	spectrum (1)		56.38 ± 0.01	56.62 ± 0.06	**0.02 ± 0.01**	0.01 ± 0.01
	spectrum (2)		53.12 ± 0.01	52.29 ± 0.07	0.04 ± 0.02	**0.00 ± 0.00**
	Nascimento et al. [23]	Biorthogonal 3.7	**100.00 ± 0.00**	93.80 ± 0.03	5.10 ± 0.64	0.01 ± 0.01
		Daubechies 8	**100.00 ± 0.00**	94.40 ± 0.03	5.12 ± 0.45	0.03 ± 0.06
		Symlet 8	**100.00 ± 0.00**	96.39 ± 0.02	11.61 ± 1.55	0.01 ± 0.01
	Our design flow (fig. 9) with wavelets	Biorthogonal 3.7	99.58 ± 0.00	94.12 ± 0.04	0.15 ± 0.01	0.01 ± 0.01
		Daubechies 8	99.87 ± 0.00	95.52 ± 0.03	0.13 ± 0.02	0.01 ± 0.01
		Symlet 8	99.63 ± 0.00	95.83 ± 0.03	0.15 ± 0.02	0.02 ± 0.01
SVM, polynomial	Proposed model	--	98.92 ± 0.00	93.92 ± 0.03	3.12 ± 3.67	0.01 ± 0.02
	spectrum (1)		57.72 ± 0.01	56.95 ± 0.04	2.00 ± 0.30	0.00 ± 0.01
	spectrum (2)		56.36 ± 0.01	55.40 ± 0.04	2.24 ± 0.39	0.00 ± 0.00
	Nascimento et al. [23]	Biorthogonal 3.7	95.84 ± 0.02	91.06 ± 0.04	11.99 ± 0.33	0.01 ± 0.01
		Daubechies 8	89.48 ± 0.03	85.22 ± 0.06	13.68 ± 0.58	0.01 ± 0.02
		Symlet 8	90.14 ± 0.02	84.08 ± 0.05	11.57 ± 0.59	0.01 ± 0.01
	Our design flow (fig. 9) with wavelets	Biorthogonal 3.7	99.17 ± 0.00	92.53 ± 0.03	7.42 ± 3.84	0.02 ± 0.01
		Daubechies 8	99.14 ± 0.00	95.23 ± 0.02	10.19 ± 3.49	0.02 ± 0.01
		Symlet 8	98.85 ± 0.01	95.38 ± 0.03	9.37 ± 3.72	0.01 ± 0.02
SVM, RBF	Proposed model	--	99.05 ± 0.00	75.43 ± 0.04	0.25 ± 0.01	0.03 ± 0.01
	spectrum (1)		57.96 ± 0.01	55.69 ± 0.06	**0.02 ± 0.01**	0.01 ± 0.01
	spectrum (2)		53.79 ± 0.01	52.07 ± 0.05	**0.02 ± 0.01**	0.00 ± 0.00
	Nascimento et al. [23]	Biorthogonal 3.7	**100.00 ± 0.00**	81.32 ± 0.03	0.19 ± 0.00	0.02 ± 0.01
		Daubechies 8	**100.00 ± 0.00**	81.32 ± 0.03	0.19 ± 0.01	0.02 ± 0.01
		Symlet 8	**100.00 ± 0.00**	81.32 ± 0.03	0.19 ± 0.01	0.03 ± 0.02
	Our design flow (fig. 9) with wavelets	Biorthogonal 3.7	99.26 ± 0.00	80.30 ± 0.04	0.25 ± 0.01	0.03 ± 0.01
		Daubechies 8	99.52 ± 0.00	80.74 ± 0.03	0.24 ± 0.01	0.04 ± 0.01
		Symlet 8	99.30 ± 0.00	80.16 ± 0.04	0.25 ± 0.01	0.03 ± 0.01

Yet considering the linear kernel our proposal and method of Nascimento et al. (2013), with Symlet 8 function, were able to achieve the best accuracies. In this case, the ratio between accuracy and training time obtained with our proposal was 20 times higher than the ratio obtained using the method of Nascimento et al. (2013).

The morphological spectrum applications showed the lowest training times compared to other approaches, in all kernels. The accuracy, however, was much lower than the other techniques, in all tests. Accuracy rates are around 50%. Therefore, the use of morphological spectra as feature extractors was not able to get feasible results in this application. Although this approach could achieve the highest ratios between average accuracy and training time, it does not make sense adopting a classifier with accuracy rates around 50%, because it is almost a random result.

Figure 10 shows boxplots of performance by the approaches we evaluated. The configuration based on linear kernels achieved the best accuracy of all networks, exception of morphological spectrum. Our method are highlight. It has the best average performance with a low dispersion. In addition, our method achieves maximum precision of 100%, depending of the data set arrangement.

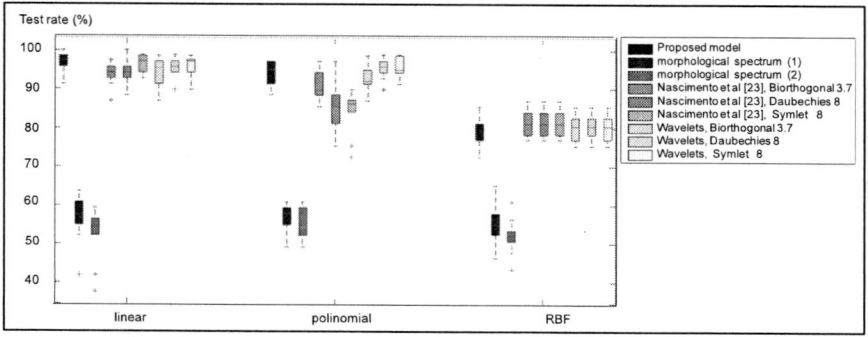

Source: The authors.

Figure 10. Boxplots of the percentage accuracy rates obtained with our proposals and the state-of-the-art techniques.

Taking into account polynomial kernels, our proposal could reach better results than the method of Nascimento et al. (2013), once we achieved sensibly higher accuracy rate. Furthermore, results got by the method of Nascimento et al. (2013) presented a considerable dispersion, depending on data set arrangement, e.g., when the Symlet 8 function is used, the results fluctuate sharply negatively, reaching a case with 72.46% of accuracy.

Regarding RBF kernels, our proposal was just slightly lower than the method of Nascimento et al. (2013). The change of morphological Decomposition by wavelets, in our design flow, obtained better results compared to all approaches, including the work of Nascimento et al. (2013).

Figure 11 shows boxplots of training times obtained by the approaches we evaluated. Regarding linear kernels, the work of Nascimento et al. (2013) could not achieve reasonable results, once its computational cost was considerably high. Furthermore, results obtained by using the approach of Nascimento et al. (2013) presented high dispersion. Nevertheless, in the best cases, the learning process consumes much more time compared to other approaches.

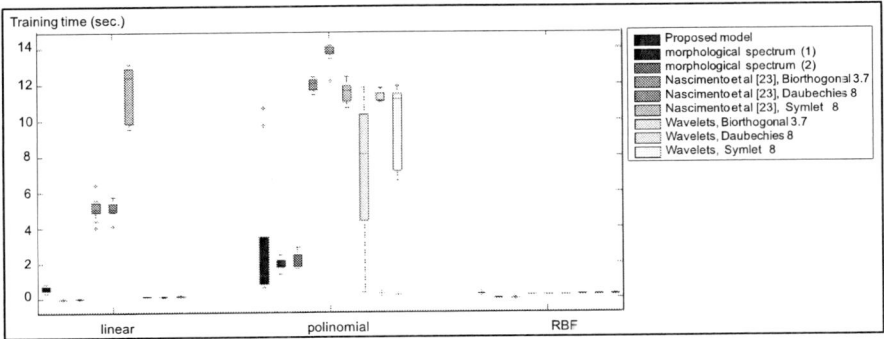

Source: The authors.

Figure 11. Boxplots of the training times of our proposal and the methods of the state-of-the-art, as estimation of computational costs.

In relation to polynomial kernels, our proposal demonstrated to have lower average computational cost, when compared to the work of Nascimento et al. (2013). Furthermore, the dispersion of our method is significantly lower when compared to Nascimento et al. (2013).

Considering RBF kernels, computational costs were sensibly low for all approaches, with very low dispersions. Hence, in these cases, learning times were stable, without abrupt changes, independently of the data set arrangement. In all evaluated kernels, the morphological spectrum obtained suitable computational costs.

CONCLUSION

We develop a methodology for detection and classification of breast mass in mammography images. Our main contribution is a class of Morphological Decomposition and it is employed on image feature description. The classification was based on neural networks based on kernels. Different types of networks were used in order to show that efficiency of Morphological Decomposition is not in function of an appropriate mapping data obtained by a particular kernel. Morphological Decomposition are able to provide excellent results in various types of neural networks and distinct learning functions.

For the experiments, we used the classification criteria for mammographic images defined according to American College of Radiology. The goal was to group the cases into three classes: normal (i.e., without cancer), benign and malignant lesion. The proposed methodology shows an average precision of 96.56%. The change of morphological Decomposition by Wavelets in design flow, caused a slight decrease in results. The best performance achieved by this approach was 95.83%. Despite minimal difference, Morphological Decomposition showed its relevance in our design flow. As closer to maximum precision more difficult is to raise the performance of a given solution. Thus, Morphological Decomposition constituted as an excellent solution. There was an increment in precision without a substantial increase in learning time.

In relation to state-of-the-art, the proposed methodology has the great advantage that not employing human segmentation both in training and use phases. This enables that the proposed work can be widely replicated in order to verify the accuracy of presented results. Furthermore, human segmentations can make the process lengthy, stressfully and more error-prone. In addition, health professionals may have difficulties in handling a computational tool in order to extract features from medical images.

The Morphological Spectrum, as an alternative to Morphological Decomposition, was a failed attempt. It is able to analyze the mass shape, however, it despises its texture. Thus, an important requirement of lesion presence study was ignored. Possibly by excluding normal cases (no mass), morphological spectrum could be successful. Our goal, however, differs from much other of state-of-the-art because we are able to not only classify between benign and malignant lesions but also to detect the presence or absence of lesion.

Our work can be extended in order to be applied to other breast types, as dense and predominant dense. In addition, our methodology can be applied to classification problems in other biomedical imaging as other cancers in which as shape as texture are essential in order to classify the anatomical abnormalities.

The proposed work was developed in order to increase chances of recovery of patients affected by breast cancer Thus, it is expected to contribute that these anomalies stopping occupying the top positions in the mortality rate of the world population. There is the expectation that the proposed system will be used in the hospital network and serve as a parameter in the detection and classification of breast cancer.

ACKNOWLEDGMENTS

The authors thank Brazil's REUNI (ref. 01/2012) for the partial financial support. The IRMA database is courtesy of Prof. Thomas M. Deserno, from the Department of Medical Informatics at RWTH Aachen University, Germany.

REFERENCES

[1] *Statistical data about breast cancer, according Brazilian Government* (in Portuguese). Available in: http://www.inca.gov.br/estimativa/2014/sintese-de-resultados-comentarios.asp. Accessed on February 2013.

[2] *U.S. Department of Health and Human Services. Obesity Among Adults in the United States - No statistically Significant Change Since 2003-2004*. Available in: http://www.cdc.gov/nchs/data/databriefs/db01.pdf. Accessed on January 2015.

[3] *U.S. Department of Health and Human Services. Prevalence of Obesity Among Adults: United States, 2011–2012*. Available in: http://www.cdc.gov/nchs/data/databriefs/db131.pdf. Accessed on January 2015.

[4] Finucane, M. M., Stevens, G. A., Cowan, M. J., Danaei, G., Lin, J. K., Paciorek, C. J., Singh, G. M., Gutierrez, H. R., Lu, Y., Bahalim, A. N., Farzadfar, F., Riley, L. M., and Ezzati, M. (2011). "National, regional, and global trends in body-mass index since 1980: systematic analysis of health examination surveys and epidemiological studies with 960 country-years and 9.1 million participants." *The Lancet* 377(9765), 557-567.

[5] Doak, C. M., Wijnhoven, T. M., Schokker, D. F., Visscher, T. L., and Seidell, J. C. (2012). "Age standardization in mapping adult overweight and obesity trends in the WHO European Region." *Obesity Reviews* 13(2), 174-191.

[6] Statistical data from OECD (Organization for Economic Co-operation and Development). Available in: http://dx.doi.org/10.1787/health-data-en. Accessed on January 2015.

[7] Costa, H., Solla, J., and Temporão, J. G. (2004). *Control of Breast Cancer. Consensus Document* (in Portuguese). Ministry of Health. National Cancer Institute.

[8] *Statistical data for breast cancer, from IARC (International Agency for Research on Cancer) of WHO (World Health Organization).* Available in: http://www.iarc.fr/en/media-centre/pr/2013/pdfs/pr223_E.pdf. Accessed on February 2013.

[9] *Prognostic Factors in Breast Cancer, according Brazilian Government* (in Portuguese). Available in: http://www.inca.gov.br/rbc/n_48/ v01/pdf/revisao.pdf. Accessed on January 2011.

[10] *Statistical data from World Health Organization.* Available in: https://apps.who.int/infobase/. Accessed on January 2015.

[11] World Health Organization. (2010). *Improving the quality and use of birth, death and cause-of-death information: guidance for a standards-based review of country practices.*

[12] Ferreira, V. A., and Magalhães, R. (2011). *Daily eating habits of obese women living in Rocinha Shantytown (Rio de Janeiro, RJ, Brazil)* (in Portuguese). Ciência Saúde Coletiva. Rio de Janeiro, June 16(6).

[13] Wells, J. C. K., Marphatia, A. A., Cole, T. J., and Mccoy, D. (2012). "Associations of Economic and Gender Inequality with Global

Obesity Prevalence: Understanding the Female Excess." *Social Science & Medicine* 75(3), 482–490.

[14] Secretary of Legislative Affairs of Ministry of Justice. *Public Records and Retrieval Public Lands* (in Portuguese). Brasilia, Brazil, 2012.

[15] *Research of IBGE (Brazilian Institute of Geography and Statistics) about household budget, 2002-2003*. Availabe in: http://www.ibge.gov.br/home/estatistica/populacao/condicaodevida/pof/2002analise/pof2002analise.pdf. Accessed on April 2009.

[16] *Research of IBGE (Brazilian Institute of Geography and Statistics) about household budget, 2008-2009*. Available in: ftp://ftp.ibge.gov.br/Indicadores_Sociais/Sintese_de_Indicadores_Sociais_2012/SIS_2012.pdf. Accessed on February 2014.

[17] Alvaredo, F., and Gasparini, L. (2015). *Handbook of Income Distribution. Chapter 9 – Recent Trends in Inequality and Poverty in Developing Countries*. Elsevier Publishing Solutions 2:697-805.

[18] Kremer, M., and Glennerster, R. (2011). *Handbook of Health Economics. Capítulo 4 – Improving Health in Developing Countries: Evidence from Randomized Evaluations*. Elsevier Publishing Solutions 2:201-315.

[19] Reydon, B. P., Fernandes, V. B., and Telles, T. S. (2015). *Land Tenure in Brazil: The Question of Regulation and Governance*. Land Use Policy 42:509-516.

[20] E. T. Paulino. (2015). The agricultural, Environmental and Socio-Political Repercussions of Brazil's Land Governance System. *Land Use Policy 36*, 134-144.

[21] *Developing Country Regions, by FAO* (Food and Agriculture Organization of the United Nations). Available in: http://www.fao.org/docrep/003/t0800e/t0800e07.htm. Accessed on January 2015.

[22] Juhl, J. H., Crummy, A. B., and Kuhlman, J. E. (1998). *Essentials of radilogic imaging*. Seventh edition. Lippincott Williams and Wilkins: New York.

[23] Nascimento, M. Z., Martins, A. S., Neves, L. A., Ramos, R. P., Flores, L. E., and Carrijo, G. A. (2013). "Classification of masses in

mammographic image using wavelet domain features and polynomial classifier." *Expert Systems with Applications* 40(1), 6213–6221.

[24] Rouhi, R., Jafarib, M., Kasaeic, S., and Keshavarziana, P. (2015). "Benign and malignant breast tumors classification based on region growing and CNN segmentation." *Expert Systems with Applications* 42(3), 990–1002.

[25] Tahmasbi, A., Saki, F., and Shokouhi, S. B. (2011). "Classification of benign and malignant masses based on Zernike moments." *Computers in Biology and Medicine* 41(1), 726–735.

[26] Saki, F., Tahmasbi, A., Soltanian-Zadeh, H., and Shokouhi, S. B. (2013). "Fast opposite weight learning rules with application in breast cancer diagnosis." *Computers in Biology and Medicine* 43(1), 32–41.

[27] Tahmasbi, A., Saki, F., Amirkhani, A., Mohamma, S., and Shokouhi, S. B. (2012). "Classification of Breast Masses based on Cognitive Resonance." *International Journal of Computer and Electrical Engineering* 4(3).

[28] Liu, X., and Tang, J. (2014). "Mass Classification in Mammograms Using Selected Geometry and Texture Features, and a New SVM-Based Feature Selection Method." *IEEE Systems Journal* 8(3).

[29] Wang, Z., Yu, G., Kang, Y., Zhao, Y., and Qu, Q. (2014). "Breast tumor detection in digital mammography based on extreme learning machine." *Neurocomputing* 128(27), 175–184.

[30] Pereira, D. C., Ramos, R. P., and Nascimento, M. Z. (2014). "Segmentation and detection of breast cancer in mammograms combining wavelet analysis and genetic algorithm." *Computer Methods and Programs in Biomedicine* 114(1), 88-101.

[31] Mallat, S. (1999). *A wavelet tour of signal processing*. Second edition. New York: Academic.

[32] He, Z., and Wang, Q. (2014). "Kernel Sparse Multitask Learning for Hyperspectral Image Classification with Empirical Mode Decomposition and Morphological Wavelet-Based Features." *IEEE Transactions on Geoscience and Remote Sensing* 52(8), 5150–5163.

[33] Quesada-Barriuso, P., Argüello, F., and Heras, D. B. (2014). "Spectral–Spatial Classification of Hyperspectral Images Using

Wavelets and Extended Morphological Profiles." *IEEE Journal of Selected Topics in Applied Earth Observations and Remote Sensing* 7(4), 1177–1185.

[34] *BI-RADSTM (Breast Imaging - Reporting and Data System)*. (2003). American College of Radiology. Fourth edition.

[35] Lehmann, T. M., Güld, M. O., Thies, C., Fischer, B., Spitzer, K., Keysers, D., Ney, H., Kohnen, M., Schubert, H., and Wein, B. (2004). "Content-based image retrieval in medical applications." *Methods of Information in Medicine* 43(4), 354–361.

[36] Suckling, J., Parker, J. Dance, D., Astley, S., Hutt, I., Boggis, C., Ricketts, I., Stamatakis, E., Cerneaz, N., Kok, S., Taylor, P., Betal, D., and Savage, J. (1994). "The mammographic image analysis society digital mammogram database exerpta medica." *International Congress Series* 1069, 375–378.

[37] Heath, M D., and Bowyer, K.W. (2000). *Mass detection by relative image intensity, 5th International Conference on Digital Mammography*. Medical Physics Publishing (Madison, WI): Toronto, Canada, ISBN 1-930524-00-5.

[38] Soille, P. (2004). *Morphological Image Analysis Principles and Applications*. Springer-Verlag.

[39] Hänni, M., Banos, I. L., Nilsson, S., Häggroth, L., and Smedby, O. (1999). "Quantitation of atherosclerosis by magnetic resonance imaging and 3D morphology operators." *Magnetic Resonance Imaging* 4:585–591.

[40] Thanh, N. D., Binh, V. D., Mi, N. T. T., and Giang, N. T. (2007). "A Robust Document Skew Estimation Algorithm using Mathematical Morphology." *IEEE International Conference on Tools with Artificial Intelligence*, Patras, Greece, 496–503.

[41] Santos, W. P., Mello, C. A. B., and Oliveira, A. L. I. (2011). "Mathematical Morphology." In *Digital Document Analysis and Processing*, 159-192. New York: Nova Science.

[42] Hagan, M. T., Demuth, H. B., and Beale, M. H. (1996). *Neural network design*, Boston, MA: PWS Publishing.

[43] Powell, M. J. D. (1977). "Restart procedures for the conjugate gradient method." *Mathematical Programming* 12, 241–254.
[44] Notay, Y. (2000). "Flexible conjugate gradients." *SIAM Journal on Scientific Computing* 22 (4): 1444. doi:10.1137/ S1064827599362314.
[45] Scales, L. E. (1985). *Introduction to non-linear optimization*, New York: Springer-Verlag.
[46] Battiti, R. (1992). "First and second order methods for learning: between steepest descent and newton's method." *Neural Computation* 4(2), 141–166.
[47] Riedmiller, M., and Braun, H. (1993). "A direct adaptive method for faster backpropagation learning: the {RPROP} algorithm." In *Proceedings of the IEEE International Conference on Neural Networks (ICNN)*, San Francisco (1993), 586–591.
[48] Moller, M. F. (1993). "Original contribution: a scaled conjugate gradient algorithm for fast supervised learning." *Neural Network* 6(4), 525–533.
[49] Huang, G. B., Zhou, H., Ding, X., and Zhang, R. (2012). "Extreme learning machine for regression and multiclass classification." *IEEE Transactions on Systems, Man, and Cybernetics* 42(2), 513 – 529.
[50] Chih-Chung, C., and Chih-Jen, L. (2011). "LIBSVM: A library for support vector machines." *ACM Transactions on Intelligent Systems and Technology*, Available in: http://www.csie.ntu.edu. tw/~cjlin/libsvm/.
[51] Santana, M. A., Pereira, J. M. S., Silva, F. L., Lima, N. M., Sousa, F. N., Arruda, G. M. S., Lima, R. C. F., Silva, W. W. A., and Santos, W. P. (2018). "Breast cancer diagnosis based on mammary thermography and extreme learning machines." *Research on Biomedical Engineering* 34(1):45-53. Epub March 05, 2018. https://dx.doi.org/10.1590/2446-4740.05217.
[52] Rodrigues, A. L., Santana, M. A., Azevedo, W. W., Bezerra, R. S., Santos, W. P., and Lima, R. C. F. (2018). "Seleção de Atributos para Apoio ao Diagnóstico do Câncer de Mama Usando Imagens Termográficas, Algoritmos Genéticos e Otimização por Enxame de

Partículas." Paper presented at *II Simpósio de Inovação em Engenharia Biomédica (SABIO 2018)*, Recife, Brazil. ["Attribute Selection to Support Breast Cancer Diagnosis Using Thermographic Imaging, Genetic Algorithms, and Particle Swarm Optimization." Paper presented at *II Biomedical Engineering Innovation Symposium (SABIO 2018)*, Recife, Brazil.]

[53] Lima, S. M. L, Silva-Filho, A. G., and Santos, W. P. (2016). "Detection and classification of masses in mammographic images in a multi-kernel approach." *Computer Methods and Programs in Biomedicine* 134:11-29. doi: 10.1016/j.cmpb.2016.04.029.

[54] Azevedo, W. W., Lima, S. M. L., Fernandes, I. M. M., Rocha, A. D. D., Cordeiro, F. R., Silva-Filho, A. G., and Santos, W. P. (2015). "Morphological extreme learning machines applied to detect and classify masses in mammograms" Paper presented at *2015 International Joint Conference of Neural Networks (IJCNN)*, Killarney, Ireland.

[55] Cordeiro, F. R., Santos, W. P., and Silva-Filho, A. G. (2016). "A semi-supervised fuzzy GrowCut algorithm to segment and classify regions of interest of mammographic images." *Expert Systems with Applications* 65(2016):116-126.

[56] de Lima, S. M. L., Silva, W. W. A., Cordeiro, F. R., da Silva-Filho, A. G., and Santos, W. P. (2015). "Features Extraction Employing Fuzzy-Morphological Decomposition for Detection and Classification of Mass on Mammograms" Paper presented at the *Engineering in Medicine and Biology Conference Management System (EMBC)*, Milan.

[57] Azevedo, W. W., Lima, S. M. L., Fernandes, I. M. M., Rocha, A. D. D., Cordeiro, F. R., Da Silva-Filho, A. G., and Dos Santos, W. P. (2015). "Fuzzy Morphological Extreme Learning Machines to detect and classify masses in mammograms" Paper presented at *2015 IEEE International Conference on Fuzzy Systems (FUZZIEEE)*, Istanbul.

[58] De Lima, S. M. L., Da Silva-Filho, A. G., and dos Santos, W. P. (2014). "A methodology for classification of lesions in mammographies using Zernike Moments, ELM and SVM Neural

Networks in a multi-kernel approach" Paper presented at *2014 IEEE International Conference on Systems, Man and Cybernetics (SMC)*, San Diego.

[59] Cordeiro, F. R., Lima, S. M. L., Silva-Filho, A. G., and Santos, W. P. (2012). "Segmentation of Mammography by Applying Extreme Learning Machine in Tumor Detection" Paper presented at the *International Conference on Intelligent Data Engineering and Automated Learning (IDEAL)*, Natal, Brazil.

[60] Lima, S. M. L., and Oliveira, S. C. 2010. "Computational Evaluation of Tumor Dimensions in Medical Images of Breast Cancer" Paper presented at *XXII Congresso Brasileiro de Engenharia Biomédica (CBEB)*, Tiradentes, Brazil.

In: Understanding a Cancer Diagnosis
Editors: W. P. dos Santos et al.
ISBN: 978-1-53617-520-2
© 2020 Nova Science Publishers, Inc.

Chapter 3

BREAST LESIONS CLASSIFICATION IN FRONTAL THERMOGRAPHIC IMAGES USING INTELLIGENT SYSTEMS AND MOMENTS OF HARALICK AND ZERNIKE

*Maíra Araújo de Santana[1],
Jessiane Mônica Silva Pereira[2],
Rita de Cássia Fernandes de Lima[3]
and Wellington Pinheiro dos Santos[3],**

[1]Department of Biomedical Engineering,
Federal University of Pernambuco, Recife, Brazil
[2]Department of Computer Engineering, University of Pernambuco, Recife, Brazil
[3]Department of Mechanical Engineering,
Federal University of Pernambuco, Recife, Brazil

---

* Corresponding Author's Email: wellington.santos@ufpe.br.

Abstract

Breast cancer is the most common type of cancer. It is also the most responsible for women deaths from cancer worldwide. Early detection of cancer is pointed as the main strategy to reduce mortality rates associated to the disease. Breast thermography is being considered as a promising auxiliary tool for breast cancer identification, since it provides physiological information, which commonly start at initial stages of the disease. Given the clinical variability, the diagnosis becomes a difficult task, which leads to misclassification or to the need of invasive and more complex procedures, in many clinical cases. To overcome this challenge, many groups are investing on pattern recognition techniques to support medical assessment. In this chapter, the authors verified the use of Multilayer Perceptron (MLP), Support Vector Machines (SVM), bayesian networks, search trees methods, and, specially, different configuration of Extreme Learning Machines (ELM) to classify breast lesions in thermographic images. Haralick and Zernike moments were used to caracterize the images. From this study, the authors achieved accuracy up to 95.56%, with kappa statistic around 0.93.

Keywords: breast cancer, breast thermography, Haralick moments, Zernike moments, learning machine, artificial neural networks, extreme learning machines

Introduction

Breast cancer is the most common type of cancer among women all over the world. Even presenting a good prognosis in most cases, this disease is still responsible for the greatest mortality rate from cancer in female population [1, 2, 3]. This rate is even greater for low income countries [2]. According to the World Health Organization (WHO), the early detection of cancer, which means detecting in its initial stages, is the key to reduce these numbers [3].

Nowadays, thermography technique is being used in some coutries as an auxiliary tool for breast cancer identification [4]. This method is based on the image acquisition through an infrared camera, showing the temperature distribution of the region of interest. Camera general operation consists in capturing the infrared radiation emitted by the region's surface. For this technique, there is no need for invasive procedures nor exposition to ionizing radiation. Thermographic assessment provides physiological information caused by diseases from the temperature distribution in the region. When there are cancer cells, their high metabolism increases blood flow, thus increasing the temperature in the damaged region. These physiological effects may precede in up to 10 years any anatomical change (masses and lumps) [4]. Breast thermography is already being used as a screening tool in some coutries and given its portability and low cost, it has a great potential to spread worldwide, specially to places of difficult access and low income countries.

In medical imaging field, many studies discuss the challenge of interpreting and establishing a diagnosis based on different image techniques [5, 6, 7, 8, 9, 10, 11, 12, 13, 14]. The variability of clinical cases is mainly responsible for this challenge. Since each human body is different, and diseases behave differently in each person, image diagnosis becomes an extremely hard task for health professionals.

Considering that, some groups are investing on the study of computational systems, such as artificial intelligence tools, to support specialists decision-making related to image diagnosis [5, 6, 9, 12, 13, 14]. In this way, Aguiar Junior et al. (2013) [6] achieved around 75% of accuracy in the identification of lesions in breast thermographic images, using multilayer perceptron as an intelligent classifier. Resmini et al. (2012) [12], on the other hand, achieved na accuracy close to 90% using other classifiers (SVM, KNN e Naive Bayes) to detect breast lesion. In the study of Belfort et al. (2015) [9], they proposed a detection method using SVM, from which they obtained an accuracy around 66%.

The method proposed in this chapter aims to assess the performance of different classifiers, especially the Extreme Leaning Machine (ELM), in differentiating types of breast lesions in thermographic images.

This chapter is organized in four sections. Initially, the authors present the materials and methods used in the study, then, they show and discuss the obtained results, and in the last section you will find some conclusions and findings from the approach.

MATERIALS AND METHODS

Figure 1 shows a diagram of the proposed method. Each step is further described in the following sections.

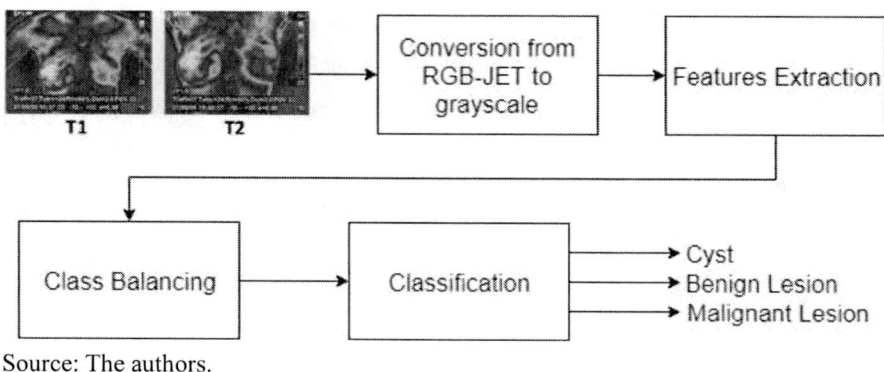

Source: The authors.

Figure 1. Brief diagram of the proposed method.

Database

This study uses thermography images acquired by a FLIR, model S45, infrared camera. The access to the images was possible through a comparison with the research group on breast thermography from the Department of Mechanical Engineering of Federal University of Pernambuco. For each patient, the group acquired eight images in different positions. Two of the images were from the frontal view of both breasts (T1 and T2), for T1 patients must be with arms down, then, they put their arms down to acquire T2 image. Another pair of images was from the frontal view of each breast individually (MD and ME). The remaining images were from the lateral view of each breast individually, being two images from the external lateral (LEMD and LEME) and two images from the internal lateral (LIMD and LIME). Further information about the acquisition process and the acquired images may be found in Oliveira (2012) [15]. This chapter presents a study where they use only the frontal images of both breasts, T1 and T2, since this condition favor the visualization of the entire breasts.

The images database was also organized according to the diagnosis previously established based on the methods commonly used in clinical practice (mammography, ultrasound, clinical exam and biopsy) [16]. This study used images where there was a cystic lesion, a benign lesion or a malignant lesion, since the main goal was to assess the method efficiency to classify the images in their respective lesion class. In other words, the authors main goal here was to identify patterns to differentiate the breast lesions. A total of 270 images was used in the experiments, being 73 of cyst, 121 of benign lesion e 76 of malignant lesion.

Features Extraction

Before the features extraction, the images were converted from RGB-JET to grayscale. Since the thermographic images use the pseudocoloring technique, where each color actually represents a value of temperature, the authors performed a conversion where the brightest colors in grayscale indicate spots with the highest temperature, and vice versa.

This approach proposes the use of Haralick moments and Zernike moments as features extractors to generate the features vectors to represent each image. The Haralick moments extract information related to image texture based on the assessment of the probability of occurence of grayscale combinations [17]. The Zernike moments, however, extract shape-related information [18].

The authors built 3 datasets based on different combinations of Haralick and Zernike descriptors. In each dataset the images were represent in a different way. In the first dataset, the authors represented the images using only Haralick moments, for the second one, they used only Zernike moments and the third dataset was built from the combination of both descriptors. All the experiments presented in this chapter were performed for each of the dataset, individually, in order to assess different methods to represent the images.

Given the difference between the amount of image in each class, the authors performed a class balancing step right after the features extraction. The balancing was performed according to the approach described in Lima, Silva-Filho and Santos (2015), where synthetic instances are created based on the linear combination of real instances [19]. Different amount of instances per group may lead to misclassification, since the algorithm may favor the class with more instances.

Classification

The classification phase was divided into 2 parts. As mentioned before, the authors performed all the experiments for three different conditions of images representation: using only Haralick moments, only Zernike moments and the combination of both extractors. They also used percentage split as test mode to create the training and testing data, so the entire dataset was splitted into 66% for train and the remaining for test.

In the first classification phase, the authors used the Extreme Learning Machine (ELM) to perform classification. For this step, they used the GNU Octave environment, version 4.0.3 [20]. ELM is a training approach for single hidden layer feedforward networks that was first proposed to overcome some issues from other approaches, such as the presence of local minima, network over-training and time-consuming learning. Studies point out advantages of ELM regarding its versatility, its performance on solving multiclass problems and its lower computational complexity, even being a nonlinear method [8, 21]. For this study, the authors tested different configurations for the number of neurons in the hidden layer and kernel function of ELM, in order to assess the best configuration. The number of neurons in the hidden layer are specially important in nonlinear problems, in general, the network adjustment increases with the amount of neurons. The authors tested five configurations for the hidden layer: with 100, 200, 300, 400 and 500 neurons. The kernel function is also essential to define the decision boundary to solve a classification challenge. For this study, linear, polynomial and radial basis function (RBF) kernels were tested. For the polynomial kernel, the study also proposes to assess performance for different exponents (p), varying from exponent 2 to 5.

In the second part of the experiments proposed in this chapter, the best ELM configuration was compared to the classification performance of widely used algorithms. The authors tested the algorithms Bayes Net, Naïve Bayes, Support Vector Machine (SVM), Multilayer Perceptron (MLP), J48, Random Forest and Random Tree. This second set of experiments was performed using the Waikato Environment fo Knowledge Analysis (WEKA), version 3.8.1, developed at the University of Waikato, New Zealand [22].

The results analysis was based on the accuracy, kappa statistic and confusion matrix. Accuracy consists in the percentage of correctly classified instances. Kappa statistics shows the rate of concordance between the expected and obtained results, it has a maximum value of 1, indicating total concordance, and values close to or below 0 (zero) indicate no concordance. The confusion matrix shows in which class each instance was classified by the method, so it is possible to see the amount of correctly classified instances and where the incorrectly classified instances were actually put. All results shown in this chapter are the mean from 20 repetitions that were performed for each configuration. Moreover, the authors present the confusion matrices for the best result obtained for each database. From the confusion matrices, the authors assessed the sensibility and specificity of the method.

RESULTS AND DISCUSSION

Extreme Learning Machine (ELM)

Table 1 shows the accuracies obtained for each dataset using ELM for the lesions classification. Overall, the accuracy increased with the increase of the amount of neurons in the hidden layer. For the dataset using Haralick moments, the best accuracy was of 76.02% and was found with linear kernel and 500 neurons. When using the dataset from Zernike moments, the authors obtained an significant increase in accuracy, if compared to the previous dataset. For Zernike dataset, the maximum accuracy was of 91.06% was found when using polynomial kernel of exponent 2 and 500 neurons in the hidden layer. For the dataset resulted from the combination of both extractors, the configuration using linear kernel and 500 neurons achieved 95.53% of accuracy.

Table 1. ELM performance regarding accuracy for each dataset

Dataset	Kernel	Neurons in hidden layer				
		100	200	300	400	500
Haralick	Linear	67.48%	69.51%	71.54%	73.98%	76.02%
	Polinomial (p = 2)	66.26%	71.95%	72.36%	72.76%	73.17%
	Polinomial (p = 3)	67.89%	70.73%	69.11%	71.54%	73.98%
	Polinomial (p = 4)	67.07%	71.54%	69.51%	71.95%	72.36%
	Polinomial (p = 5)	67.07%	68.70%	71.95%	72.36%	71.95%
	RBF	58.13%	60.98%	63.82%	63.82%	66.26%
Zernike	Linear	85.77%	86.18%	86.59%	86.59%	86.99%
	Polinomial (p = 2)	83.33%	86.59%	90.24%	90.65%	91.06%
	Polinomial (p = 3)	80.89%	87.40%	86.18%	88.21%	89.02%
	Polinomial (p = 4)	78.05%	82.52%	86.99%	88.21%	86.59%
	Polinomial (p = 5)	73.98%	81.71%	83.74%	87.40%	86.99%
	RBF	81.71%	84.15%	86.18%	86.99%	87.80%
Haralick and Zernike	Linear	88.62%	93.50%	93.90%	95.12%	95.53%
	Polinomial (p = 2)	84.96%	89.84%	90.65%	91.06%	92.68%
	Polinomial (p = 3)	80.49%	91.06%	89.02%	92.28%	91.06%
	Polinomial (p = 4)	82.93%	85.77%	87.80%	89.43%	91.06%
	Polinomial (p = 5)	76.83%	88.62%	84.55%	88.21%	88.21%
	RBF	78.46%	81.71%	88.21%	89.43%	89.43%

Table 2. ELM performance regarding kappa statistics for each dataset

Dataset	Kernel	Neurons in hidden layer				
		100	200	300	400	500
Haralick	Linear	0.51	0.54	0.57	0.61	0.64
	Polynomial (p = 2)	0.49	0.58	0.58	0.59	0.60
	Polynomial (p = 3)	0.52	0.56	0.54	0.57	0.61
	Polynomial (p = 4)	0.51	0.57	0.54	0.58	0.58
	Polynomial (p = 5)	0.51	0.53	0.58	0.58	0.58
	RBF	0.37	0.41	0.46	0.46	0.49
Zernike	Linear	0.79	0.79	0.80	0.80	0.80
	Polynomial (p = 2)	0.75	0.80	0.85	0.86	0.87
	Polynomial (p = 3)	0.71	0.81	0.79	0.82	0.84
	Polynomial (p = 4)	0.67	0.74	0.80	0.82	0.80
	Polynomial (p = 5)	0.61	0.73	0.76	0.81	0.80
	RBF	0.73	0.76	0.79	0.80	0.82
Haralick and Zernike	Linear	0.83	0.90	0.91	0.93	0.93
	Polynomial (p = 2)	0.77	0.85	0.86	0.86	0.89
	Polynomial (p = 3)	0.71	0.86	0.84	0.88	0.86
	Polynomial (p = 4)	0.74	0.79	0.82	0.84	0.86
	Polynomial (p = 5)	0.65	0.83	0.77	0.82	0.82
	RBF	0.68	0.72	0.82	0.84	0.84

Regarding kappa statistics, ELM performance followed almost the same patterns from accuracy. From Table 2, it is noticed that the best results were found when using 500 neurons in the hidden layer, closely followed by the results with 400 neurons. For Haralick dataset, the linear kernel performed better than the other, achieving a kappa of 0.64. The datasets using Zernike and using the combination of Haralick and Zernike, however, overcome this result, presenting a kappa up to 0.87 and 0.93, respectively.

The results from Tables 1 and 2 may indicate that, for ELM classifier, the differentiation of breast lesion is a difficult task, since it requires a greater amount of neurons in the hidden layer. However, its solution might be easily generalized, since the good results were achieved when using less specific or complex kernel functions. The best results were obtained using kernels linear or polynomial of exponent 2. Most of the times, the worse results were achieved by the polynomial kernel of exponents 4 and 5 and when using 100 or 200 neurons in the hidden layer.

ELM *versus* Other Methods

On the second moment, the authors performed tests to compare ELM performance to the performance of others widely used classification methods. From Figures 2 to 4, it may be seen that the worse classification performance was found when using features from Haralick moments alone (Figure 2). Classification performance increased when representing the images using Zernike moments (Figure 3). However, the best performances were achieved when the authors combined the features extracted from Haralick moments and Zernike moments (Figure 4).

For the results using the dataset from Haralick descriptor, in Figure 2, the best accuracy obtained was of around 76% using ELM, the kappa statistic for this condition was close to 0.65. ELM was closely followed by MLP and Random Forest, both achieving accuracy around 70% and kappa around 0.55. The methods with the worse performance in this case were the bayesian networks, showing accuracy between 50% and 60%, and kappa statistic between 0.3 and 0.4.

From the confusion matrix in Table 3, the authors noticed more confusion between the benign lesion and cysts. There was also some confusion between benign lesion and malignant, and between malignant lesion and cyst and benign. Almost none confusion was noticed between cyst and the other groups.

When the authors used only Zernike moments to represent the images, the methods performances increased. The results in Figure 3 shows a maximum accuracy around 90% and kappa achieving more than 0.85 for this situation. One more time this best result was found when using ELM method for classification. The methods MLP, Random Forest and SVM also showed good performance, with accuracy between 75% and 85%, and kappa statistic varying from 0.65 to 0.75. The worst result was from J48, which achieved almost 60% of accuracy and kappa close to 0.4.

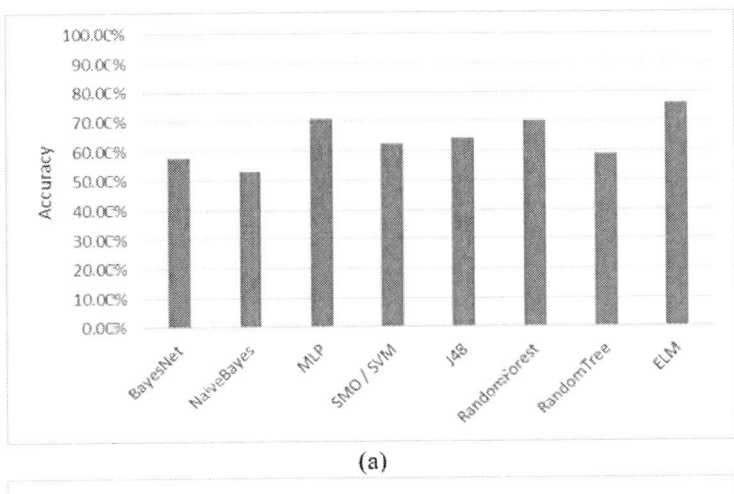

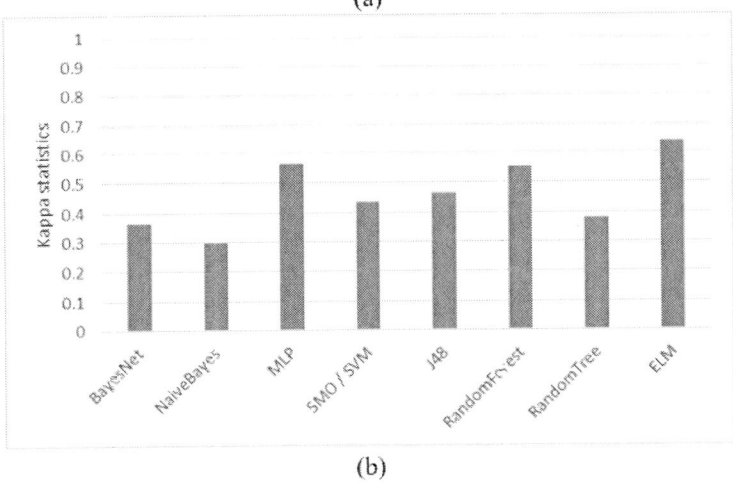

Source: The authors.

Figure 2. Classifiers performance for the dataset using Haralick moments. In (a) are the results for accuracy, while in (b) are the kappa statistics results.

Table 3. Confusion matrix for the best result using the dataset from Haralick moments

cyst	benign lesion	malignant lesion	
58	1	1	Cyst
13	41	6	benign lesion
5	4	51	malignant lesion

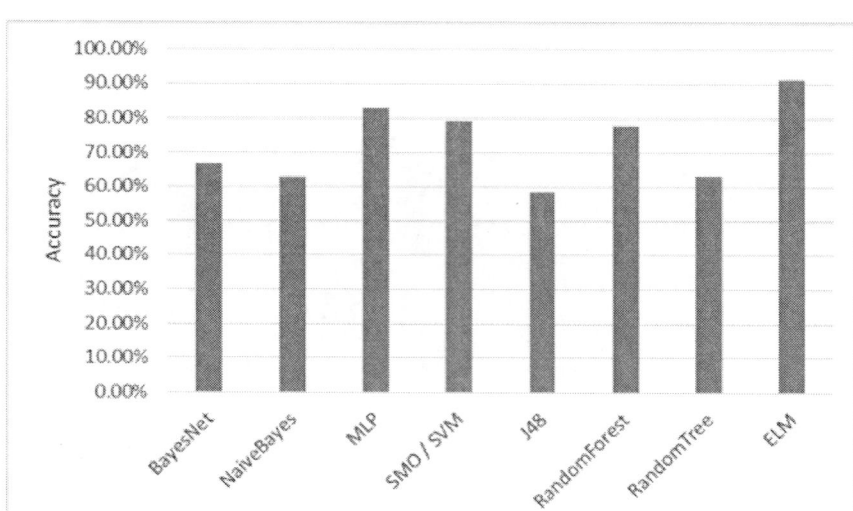

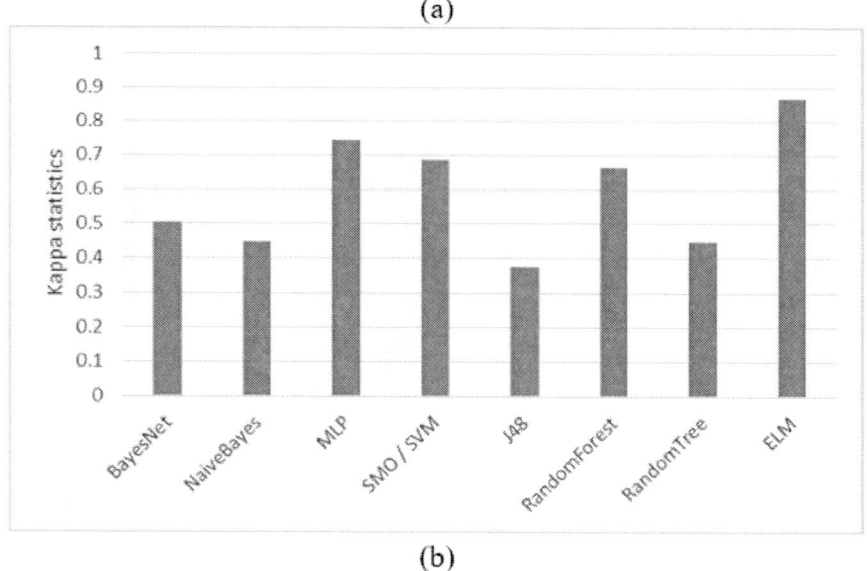

Source: The authors.

Figure 3. Classifiers performance for the dataset using Zernike moments. In (a) are the results for accuracy, while in (b) are the kappa statistics results.

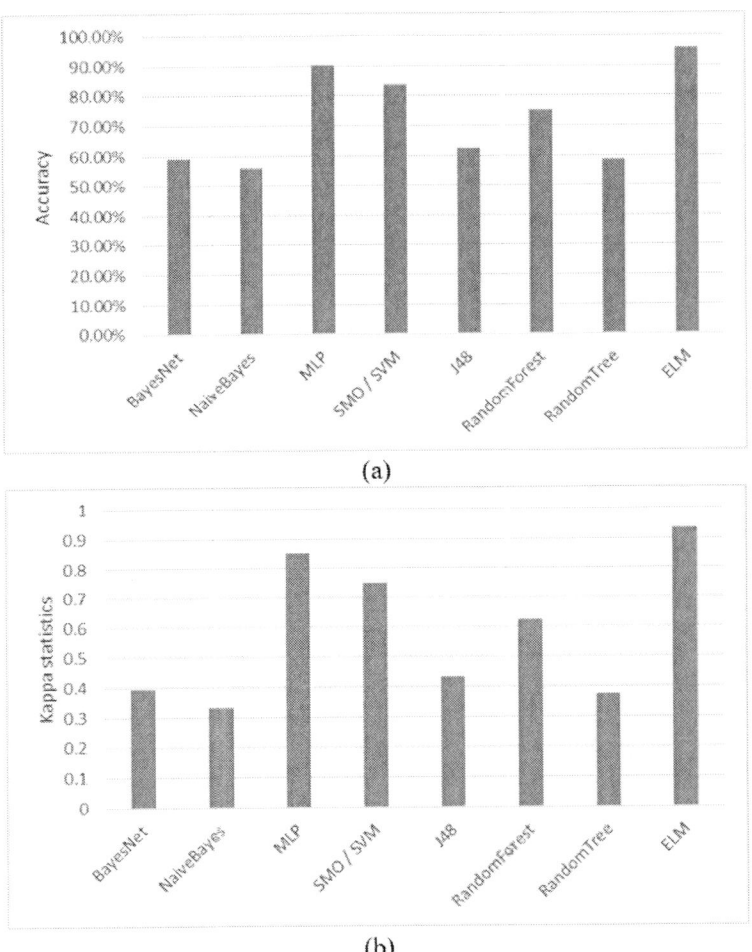

Source: The authors.

Figure 4. Classifiers performance for the dataset using the combination of Haralick and Zernike moments. In (a) are the results for accuracy, while in (b) are the kappa statistics.

For the confusion matrix obtained from the best performance using the dataset from Zernike moments (Table 4), the authors noticed a decrease in confusion between all groups. There was no confusion between the class cyst and the others classes of lesions and there was almost none confusion between malignant class and the others. Nevertheless, there was still confusion between benign lesion and the other types of lesions.

Table 4. Confusion matrix for the best result using the dataset from Zernike moments

cyst	benign lesion	malignant lesion	
60	0	0	Cyst
4	49	7	benign lesion
0	1	59	malignant lesion

Table 5. Confusion matrix for the best result using the dataset from the combination of Haralick and Zernike moments

cyst	benign lesion	malignant lesion	
59	1	0	Cyst
2	53	5	benign lesion
0	0	60	malignant lesion

Regarding the experiments using the dataset built from the combination of Haralick and Zernike moments (Figure 4), they showed the best results overall. In this situation, ELM reaching more than 95% of accuracy and around 0.90 of kappa statistic. MLP achieved the second best result (accuracy of 90% and kappa around 0.85) and was closely followed by SVM, with accuracy close to 85% and kappa above 0.75. In this scenario, the bayesian networks presented the worst performance, with accuracy below 60% and kappa statistic below 0.4. Average results were obtained by the search trees (J48, Random Tree and Random Forest).

Table 5 shows the confusion matrix for the situation where the authors combined Haralick and Zernike features. From the matrix, there was also an improvement regarding the amount of confusion between classes when using this dataset. There was no confusion between malignant lesion and the others nor cyst and the others. Even though there is still confusion for the benign lesion class, it was lower than for the previous datasets.

CONCLUSION

Overall, the confusion rates may indicate that benign lesions are harder to differentiate from the others, while cysts are much easily differentiated.

From the confusion matrices, the authors assessed the sensitivity and specificity rates of the best results. Using this approach, the authors achieved a sensitivity of 96.72% to identify cysts, 98.15% for benign lesion and 92.31% for malignant lesion. Regarding specificity, the method showed an value of 99.12% for cystic lesion, 94.44% for benign and 100% for malignant lesion.

From the results presented in this chapter, it was shown that both texture and shape information are relevant to classify different types of lesions. Furthermore, the results showed a major importance of the image shape to differentiate breast lesions in thermographic images.

Regarding the different methods of classification, results showed ELM, MLP and SVM overcome the other methods. Morover, the ELM showed to be an efficient tool for the classification of breast lesions in breast thermographic images, when acquired in frontal position. The results presented in this chapter are promising, considering that this algorithm performance was better than of the other methods applied to the datasets.

Future studies may optimize the results obtained from this approach, thus improving the identification of benign lesions and the overall breast lesion classification.

ACKNOWLEDGMENTS

The authors thank to Coordenação de Aperfeiçoamento de Pessoal de Nível Superior (CAPES), Brazil and to Fundação de Amparo à Ciência e Tecnologia de Pernambuco (FACEPE), Brazil for the support in the research.

REFERENCES

[1] American Cancer Society. 2019. *Cancer Facts & Figures 2019*. Atlanta: Global Headquarters.

[2] Instituto Nacional de Câncer José Alencar Gomes da Silva. 2015. *Diretrizes para a Detecção Precoce do Câncer de Mama no Brasil.* [*Guidelines for the Early Detection of Breast Cancer in Brazil*] Rio de Janeiro: INCA.

[3] World Health Organization. 2018. *Early Detection. Cancer control: knowledge into action: WHO guide for effective programmes.* Geneva: WHO.

[4] Etehadtavakol, M., and Ng, E. Y. K. 2013. "Breast Thermography as a Potential Non-Contact Method in the Early Detection of Cancer: A Review." *Journal of Mechanics in Medicine and Biology* 13(2):1330001. doi: 10.1142/S0219519413300019.

[5] Acharya, U. R., Ng, E. Y. K., Tan, J.-H., and Sree, S. V. 2012. "Thermography Based Breast Cancer Detection Using Texture Features and Support Vector Machine." *Journal of Medical Systems* 36(3):1503-10.

[6] Aguiar Junior, P. S., Belfort, C. N. S., Silva, A. C., Diniz, P. H. B., Lima, R. C. F., Conci, A., and Paiva, A. C. 2013. "Detecção de Regiões Suspeitas de Lesão na Mama em Imagens Térmicas Utilizando Spatiogram e Redes Neurais." ["Detection of Suspended Regions de Lesão na Mama in Thermal Using Spatiogram and Neural Networks."] *Cadernos de Pesquisa* 20(2):56-63.

[7] Andrade, M. K. S., Santana, M. A., and Santos, W. P. 2018. "Avaliação do Desempenho de Classificadores Inteligentes na Detecção da Doença de Alzheimer em Imagens de Ressonância Magnética Utilizando Extratores de Forma e Textura" ["Assessment of the Performance of Intelligent Classifiers in the Detection of Alzheimer's Disease in Magnetic Resonance Imaging Using Extractors of Shape and Texture."] Paper presented at the *II Simpósio de Inovação em Engenharia Biomédica (SABIO 2018)*, Recife, Brazil.

[8] Azevedo, W. W., Lima, S. M. L., Fernandes, I. M. M., Rocha, A. D. D., Cordeiro, F. R., Silva-Filho, A. G., and Santos, W. P. 2015. "Morphological extreme learning machines applied to detect and classify masses in mammograms" Paper presented at *2015*

International Joint Conference of Neural Networks (IJCNN), Killarney, Ireland.

[9] Belfort, C. N. S., Silva, A. C., and Paiva, A. C. 2015. "Detecção de lesões em imagens termográficas de mama utilizando Índice de Similaridade de Jaccard e Artificial Crawlers" ["Detection of lesions in breast thermographic images using Jaccard Similarity Index and Artificial Crawlers"] Paper presented at the *XV Workshop de Informática Médica*, Recife, Brazil.

[10] Cheng, H. D., Shi, X. J., Min, R., Hu, L. M., Cai, X. P., and Du, H. N. 2005. "Approaches for automated detection and classification of masses in mammograms." *Pattern Recognition* 39(2006):646-668.

[11] Cordeiro, F. R., Santos, W. P., and Silva-Filho, A. G. 2016. "A semi-supervised fuzzy GrowCut algorithm to segment and classify regions of interest of mammographic images." *Expert Systems with Applications* 65(2016):116-126.

[12] Resmini, R., Conci, A., Borchartt, T. B., Lima, R. C. F., Montenegro, A. A., and Pantaleão, C. A. 2012. "Diagnóstico Precoce de Doenças Mamárias Usando Imagens Térmicas e Aprendizado de Máquina." *Revista Eletrônica do Alto Vale de Itajaí* 1(1):55-67.

[13] Rodrigues, A. L., Santana, M. A., Azevedo, W. W., Bezerra, R. S., Santos, W. P., and Lima, R. C. F. 2018. "Seleção de Atributos para Apoio ao Diagnóstico do Câncer de Mama Usando Imagens Termográficas, Algoritmos Genéticos e Otimização por Enxame de Partículas" ["Selection of Attributes to Support Breast Cancer Diagnosis Using Thermographic Images, Genetic Algorithms and Particle Swarm Optimization"]. Paper presented at *II Simpósio de Inovação em Engenharia Biomédica (SABIO 2018)*, Recife, Brazil.

[14] Santana, M. A., Pereira, J. M. S., Silva, F. L., Lima, N. M., Sousa, F. N., Arruda, G. M. S., Lima, R. C. F., Silva, W. W. A., and Santos, W. P. 2018. "Breast cancer diagnosis based on mammary thermography and extreme learning machines." *Research on Biomedical Engineering* 34(1):45-53. Epub. March 05, 2018. https://dx.doi.org/10.1590/2446-4740.05217.

[15] Oliveira, M. M. 2012. *Desenvolvimento de protocol e construção de um aparato mecânico para padronização da aquisição de imagens termográficas de mama* [*Protocol development and construction of a mechanical apparatus for standardizing the acquisition of breast thermographic images*]. PhD diss., Federal University of Pernambuco.

[16] Dourado Neto, H. M. 2014. "*Segmentação e análise automática de termogramas: um método auxiliar na detecção do câncer de mama.*" [*"Segmentação e análise automática de termogramas: um método auxiliar na detecção do câncer de mama."*] PhD diss., Federal University of Pernambuco.

[17] Haralick, R. M., Shanmugam, K., and Dinstein, I. 1973. "Textural Features for Image Classification." *IEEE Transactions on Systems, Man, and Cybernetics* 3(6):610-621.

[18] Kan, C., and Srinath, M. D. (2001). "Combined Features of Cubic-B-Spline Wavelet Moments and Zernike Moments for Invariant Character Recofnition." Paper presented at *IEEE International Conference on Information Technology: Coding and Computing (ITCC'01)*, USA.

[19] Lima, S. M. L, Silva-Filho, A. G., and Santos, W. P. 2016. "Detection and classification of masses in mammographic images in a multi-kernel approach." *Computer Methods and Programs in Biomedicine* 134:11-29. doi: 10.1016/j.cmpb.2016.04.029.

[20] Eaton, J. W., Bateman, D., Hauberg, S., and Wehbring, R. 2018. "*GNU Octave: A high-level interactive language for numerical computations*", ed. 4. Maryland, USA.

[21] Huang, G., Zhou, H., Ding, X., and Zhang, R. "Extreme Learning Machine for Regression and Multiclass Classification." *IEEE Transactions on Systems, Man, and Cybernetics* 42(2):513-29.

[22] Hall, M., Frank, E., Holmes, G., Pfahringer, B., Reutemann, P., and Witten, I. H. 2009. "The WEKA Data Mining Software: An Update." *SIGKDD Explorations* 11(1).

In: Understanding a Cancer Diagnosis
Editors: W. P. dos Santos et al.
ISBN: 978-1-53617-520-2
© 2020 Nova Science Publishers, Inc.

Chapter 4

Lesion Detection in Breast Thermography Using Machine Learning Algorithms Without Previous Segmentation

Jessiane Mônica Silva Pereira[1],
Maíra Araújo de Santana[2],
Rita de Cássia Fernandes de Lima[3]
and Wellington Pinheiro dos Santos[2],*

[1]Polytechnique School of the University of Pernambuco, Recife, Brazil
[2]Department of Biomedical Engineering, Federal University of Pernambuco, Recife, Brazil
[3]Department of Mechanical Engineering, Federal University of Pernambuco, Recife, Brazil

---

* Corresponding Author's Email: wellington.santos@ufpe.br.

Abstract

Breast cancer in women has had a high incidence and mortality rate in the world. To reduce female mortality due to this type of cancer, early detection of breast lesions is necessary, since it increases the chance of cure, helping to make the most effective treatment decision. Among the detection devices, the most commonly used today is mammography, but it has limitations, such as difficulty in identifying some cancers without mass and cancers in dense breasts, breast susceptibility to ionizing radiation, patient discomfort due to compression of the breasts and high cost of the procedure. These problems can be overcome by associating thermographic assessment to machine learning algorithms, since thermography is a non-invasive, low-cost, non-ionizing radiation exam that does not depend on the age group or carcinogenic composition for its effectiveness. In this study, the authors proposed a method for the detection of the existence of lesions in breast thermography exams, using machine learning algorithms. The authors used Haralick and Zernike moments to perform features extraction. The best results were obtained by SVM method, achieving a maximum accuracy of 95% and a kappa statistic of more than 0.9.

Keywords: machine learning, thermography, breast cancer, early diagnosis, Haralick moments and Zernike moments

Introduction

The incidence of cancer cases is increasing worldwide. Excluding non-melanoma skin cancer, breast cancer is the most common type of cancer among women, with incidence rates of 25.2%. This disease is also one of the leading causes of cancer death in female population in low income countries [1]. The World Health Organization (WHO) states that breast cancer identified in early stages has a high cure rate [1]. Because of this, early detection of breast lesions is necessary in order to decrease patient mortality rates, increasing treatment efficiency.

There are several exams to be used in breast cancer screening, such as mammography, ultrasonography, CT scans, magnetic resonance imaging. Usually, more than one of these technique are combined to increase diagnosis accuracy. The main screening tool is mammography, which is performed by emitting x-ray beams through the breast, which achieves a film, creating an image.

However, mammography has some limitations, such as difficulty in identifying some cancers without masses, such as Paget's carcinoma [2]. This technique also has low effectiveness in dense breasts (young breasts) because of the high density of glandular tissue, which interferes with the contrast of the generated images [3, 4]. These younger breasts, are even more susceptible to the harmful effects of x-rays [5], which is one of the reasons for not recommending young people to mammographic exam. In addition, there are reports of patients regarding the discomfort caused by the exam due to breast compression during the procedure [6], and the high cost of the procedure.

In this scenario, breast thermography appears as a promising method for detecting breast lesions It is not restricted by age [3]; has low acquisition and maintenance costs compared to mammography; it is also a noninvasive exam that does not emit ionizing radiation. These images are acquired by a camera capable of capturing the infrared rays emitted by the human body [3, 7]. This emission occurs because of heat exchanges from the body surface to the environment, which is part of the normal thermoregulation process, and the largest percentage of this heat transfer occurs in the infrared range.

During the conception of most tumors, there is an increase in vascularization at the site of the lesion, increasing blood flow in that region, thereby causing an increase in temperature in the region [3]. This temperature can be observed on the surface of the breast by thermography. Since blood vessel formation occurs prior to the appearance of lumps and masses, this gives the thermography a good predictability in the detection of breast lesions. However, such temperature increase can be difficult to detect only by human observation of a thermographic image. So, the use of machine learning algorithms to analyze these images increases detection accuracy [4].

The aim of this chapter is the detection of lesions in breast thermography exams. It was performed without previous segmentation and using machine learning algorithms. In this study, Zernike [8] and Haralick [9] moments were used to extract features from thermographic images. This chapter is organized as follows: initially, the authors present some related works, then, they explain the database, followed by the proposed method and the results and discussion section. Finally, they present some conclusions and future works.

RELATED WORKS

Visual analysis of an image is often a difficult task for humans. Because of this, machine learning algorithms are constantly used in diagnosis, since they are powerful techniques to extracts information from these images and find patterns to classify complex datasets.

Osareh and Shadgar (2010) [10], used machine learning to diagnose breast cancer using two different datasets. The first one was acquired from biopsy exams, each sample was represented by 11 features (one was the patient's age and ten were cell features), they used a total of 692 samples with their respective confirmed diagnoses. The second dataset had 295 microarrays, containing the prognostic profile of 70 genes. They used the Principal Component Analysis (PCA) technique for features reduction and Signal-to-Noise Ration (SNR) filters and a Sequential Forward Selection (SFS) approach were used for features selection. After attributes selection, they applied machine learning algorithms such as Support Vector Machine (SVM), k-Nearest Neighbor (kNN) and Probabilistic Neural Network (PNN) to both datasets. Finally, they found maximum accuracies of 98.80% for the first dataset and 96.33% for the second dataset, using SVM.

Medical imaging revolutionized diagnosis, but they have not always had good imaging resolution. Imaging techniques began to be developed only in late 19th and early 20th centuries. In the case of thermography, the lack of resolution was a critical factor. The initial studies using thermographic assessment for cancer diagnosis depended a lot on camera potential, but at that time, cameras did not have a satisfactory quality. With the improvement of thermal image quality over time, people developed better detection and diagnosis systems, and created proposals for cancer identification. Some of these proposals are based on heat transfer in the lesion regio [11], while others are based on pattern recognition tools, such as the method proposed in this chapter.

Many studies require great efforts to perform segmentation stage, making the system more complex. In the paper by Wakankar and Suresh (2016) [12], they used several classifiers, such as: k-Means, Fuzzy Means and the Level Set method to segment 34 thermograms, in order to extract the region of interest (ROI). They also used color information to characterize the warmer regions. SVM was used to classify samples, achieving 91.6% of accuracy, 88.8% sensitivity and 100% specificity.

In the study from Milosevic, Jankovic and Peulic (2014) [13], the authors applied a new segmentation step after image classification. Using the techniques of minimal variance quantization, dilatation and erosion of the image, they extracted the warm region and compared it to the original image, in order to confirm if the extracted image gad the same tumor shape. According to the authors, the extracted image had almost the same shape as the tomor.

There is a wide variety of features extraction techniques [14]. In Cheng et al. (2006) [15], they used the Discrete Wavelet Transform (DWT) to obtain the initial Feature Point Image (IFI) of each segmented breast thermogram with automatic segmentation. They used 306 thermographic images from 102 and IFI features to represent the images. To reduce irrelevant features, and, consequently, the size of the set of features, MLP classifier achieved an accuracy rate of 90.48%, with sensitivity of 87.6% and specificity of 89.73%.

Features extraction techniques using texture descriptors have been successfully used in image analysis of mammograms [4, 15, 16] and thermographies [17, 18]. In the study of Pramanik, Bhattacharjee and Nasipuri (2015) [17], they computed the features based on the grayscale co-occurrence matrix, which are used to assess the effectiveness of texture information. They used SVM, Naïve Bayes and kNN classifiers to group 40 thermographic images into normal and abnormal. kNN showed the best performance, with 92.5% of accuracy.

The Database

The thermographic images used in this study were acquired by the Group of Breast Thermography from the Department of Mechanical Engineering of Federal University of Pernambuco, Brazil. The infrared camera was a FLIR camera of S45 model, which provides an image resolution of 320x240. All images were acquired under medical supervision, according to all ethical principles and using standardized protocols [19].

For each patient, they acquired breast images from eight different positions: two frontal images of both breasts, one with hands down (T1) and the other with hands up (T2); one frontal image from each breast, individually (MD, for right breast, and ME, for left breast); and four images from lateral views of each breast, being two from the external lateral view (LEMD, for right breast and LEME for left breast) and two from the internal lateral view (LIMD, for right breast and LIME for left breast). Figure 1 presents samples of images in each position.

The database has 1052 images, which were classified according to the diagnosis: cyst, benign lesion, malignant lesion or no lesion (see Table 1 for further information). All diagnoses were established after investigation using specific exams for each case, such as mammography, fine needle aspiration, ultrasonography or biopsy [20].

Methods

The proposed method follows the steps presented in Figure 2. First of all, the authors performed an images selection, then, they converted the images from RGB-JET to grayscale. Right after the conversion, they performed features extraction, followed by a class balancing step, and finally, the classification of the images in their respective group. Each of these steps is further explained in the following sections.

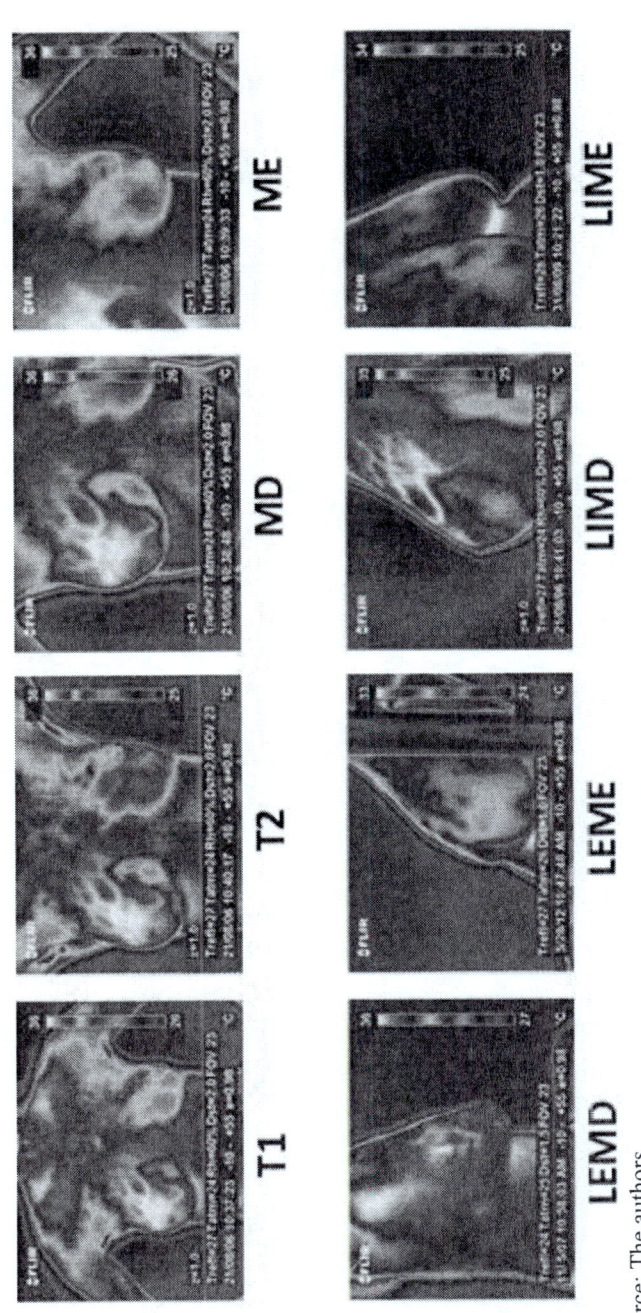

Source: The authors.

Figure 1. Samples of images acquired in a breast thermography exam.

Table 1. Amount of images per diagnosis group on database

	Diagnosis				
	Cyst	Benign lesion	Malignant lesion	No lesion	Total
Number of images	219	371	235	227	1052

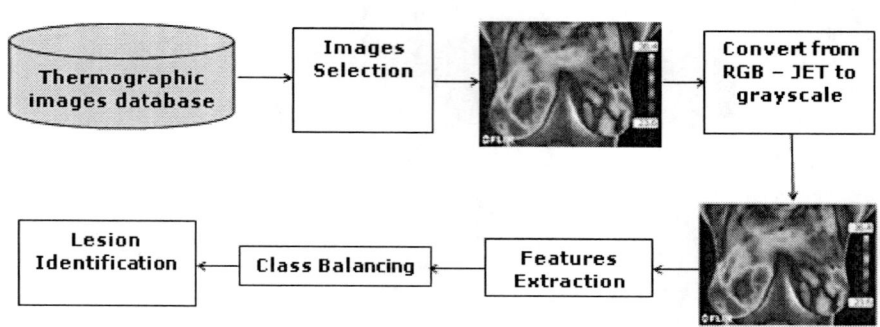

Source: The authors.

Figure 2. Diagram of the proposed method.

Images Selection

For this study, the authors combined the images of cyst, benign lesion and malignant lesion into a new class called "lesion." So they could assess system performance in identifying the presence of lesion by proposing a two-class problem, in which the image should be classified as "lesion" or "no lesion." Furthermore, the authors chose to use only T1 and T2 images, since this position provides a better visualization of the entire breasts.

In this reduced set of images, there were a total of 336 images, being 270 of the lesion class and 66 images without lesion. Samples of images from each group is shown in Figure 3.

Lesion Detection in Breast Thermography Using Machine Learning... 99

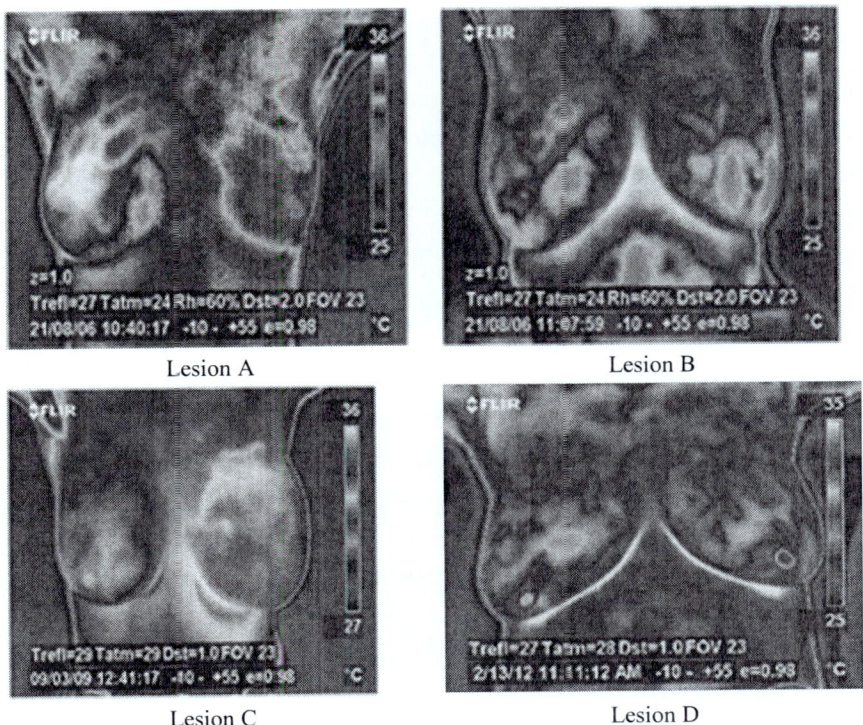

Lesion A Lesion B

Lesion C Lesion D

Source: The authors.

Figure 3. Samples of images from lesion and no lesion classes.

Preprocessing

The preprocessing consisted of only one step, converting RGB-JET to 8-bit grayscale. The conversion was necessary to standardize the information from the pseudocoloring processing, thus avoiding errors due to different color palettes used during images acquisition. In this process, the lighter shades from grayscale indicates higher temperatures, and vice versa.

Each pseudo-color in the color palette corresponds to a temperatura. You may obtain the temperature matrix of a thermographic image by performing the inverse transformation from pseudo-colors to temperature. This matrix was mapped to 0 to 255 gray levels (8 bits).

There was no use of specialized software to remove the information the camera adds to the images, such as bars, numbers and labels. Since this information is always in the same position, the authors believed that the classifiers might interpret this information as redundant and disregard it. Skipping this step decreases the duration and complexity of the entire process.

Features Extraction

The method proposed in this chapter used Haralick moments and Zernike moments to represent the thermographic images. Both descriptors are widely used to extract features from breast images [21, 22, 23, 24]. From these descriptors, the authors built three different datasets, one using only Haralick moments (104 features), another one using Zernike moments alone (64 features), and the last one combining the features extracted from both techniques (168 features).

Haralick moments provide texture-based information. Extractors of this type calculates a series of information from the image, such as entropy, correlation, variance and energy. Haralick texture features extraction process is based on the Gray Level Co-Occurrence Matrix (GLCM) and usually have a satisfactory features description, even when images have overlapping information [9, 21].

On the other hand, Zernike moments are used to recognize shape-related patterns [22, 23], so they build a mapping in a complex set of Zernike polynomials, which are orthogonal to each other. This characteristic makes possible to represent image properties without redundancy or information overlap between moments [8, 24].

Postprocessing

Such as previously described, the amount of images in each class was very different. So, to avoid biased result during training, leading to misclassification, the author performed a linear class balancing. They used a data interpolation by inserting synthetic vectors calculated from the barycenter of real instances [23]. After class balancing, each class now has 540 instances.

Classification

For classification phase, the study assessed the performance of seven classifiers: Bayes Net [25], Naïve Bayes [26], Multilayer Perceptron (MLP) [27], Support Vector Machine (SVM) [28], J48 [26], Random Forest [29, 30] and Random Tree [31, 32, 33]. All methods were tested using the Waikato Environment for Knowledge Analysis (WEKA), version 3.8, developed at the University of Waikato, New Zealand [34] using the parameters presented in Table 2. The authors used a 10-fold cross-validation method to validate the training [35].

Table 2. Configuration for each classifier

Classifier	Parameters
Bayes Net	-
Naïve Bayes	-
J48	-
SVM	Linear kernel
MLP	Hidden Layers: a*
	Learning Rate: 0.3
	Momentum: 0.2
	Iterations: 500
Random Forest	Trees: 100
Random Tree	-

*a = (nAttributes + nClasses)/2.

RESULTS AND DISCUSSION

Such as previously mentioned, the authors perfomed all tests for the three different databases. Table 3 presents the accuracy and kappa statistic results for each classification method for the dataset where the images were represented by Haralick moments alone.

For this situation, MLP performed better than the other methods, showing an accuracy of 87.68% and kappa of 0.7537 for the lesion detection task. It was closely followed by the performance of the Random Forest classifier, with 85.83% of accuracy and 0.7167 of kappa statistic. Naive Bayes performed worse than the other methods, but still achieving a moderate result: 72.22% of accuracy and 0.4444 of kappa.

Table 3. Classification performance for each method using Haralick moments for features extraction

Classifier	Accuracy (%)	Kappa statistic
Bayes Net	77.68	0.5537
Naive Bayes	72.22	0.4444
MLP	87.68	0.7537
SVM	77.96	0.5593
J48	80.37	0.6074
Random Forest	85.83	0.7167
Random Tree	79.81	0.5963

In a second moment, the images were represented by features extracted from Zernike moments. From Table 4, an increase in the best classification performance becomes clear when using Zernike moments, if compared to the condition where only Haralick moments were used for features extraction. One more time, MLP overcame the other methods, presenting an accuracy of 92.96% and kappa statistic of 0.8593. The second best performance was from Random Forest, which achieved 87.59% of accuracy and 0.7519 of kappa. The worst result for this dataset, however, was found when using Random Tree as classifier (73.33% and 0.4667). The performance of Bayes Net remained almost the same as in the previous database. There was also an increase in the results from Naïve Bayes and SVM, while J48 and Random Tree performed worse than when using features from Haralick moments.

Table 4. Classification performance for each method using Zernike moments for features extraction

Classifier	Accuracy (%)	Kappa statistic
Bayes Net	77.41	0.5481
Naive Bayes	76.94	0.5389
MLP	92.96	0.8593
SVM	84.26	0.6852
J48	76.76	0.5352
Random Forest	87.59	0.7519
Random Tree	73.33	0.4667

Table 5. Classification performance for each method using the combination of Haralick and Zernike moments for features extraction

Classifier	Accuracy (%)	Kappa statistic
Bayes Net	76.02	0.5204
Naive Bayes	71.67	0.4333
MLP	95.09	0.9019
SVM	88.33	0.7667
J48	80.65	0.6130
Random Forest	89.26	0.7852
Random Tree	74.44	0.4889

Table 6. Confusion matrix for the best result found in this study

Lesion	No lesion	
503	37	Lesion
16	524	No lesion

The authors also represented the images through the combination of both descriptors, in an attempt to improve classification. Table 5 shows the results obtained in this scenario. MLP was again responsible for the best performance overall, presenting an accuracy of 95.09% and a kappa statistic of 0.9019. A little under MLP are Random Forest and SVM classifiers, with accuracies around 89% and 88%, respectively. Such as when using only Haralick features, Naïve Bayes showed the worst performance overall, which was 71.67% of accuracy and 0.4333 of kappa, this result was even lower than the one for the first dataset.

Overall, the authors found that Random Tree and the bayesian networks showed lowest performances in almost all situations, indicating some dependency among the features. The results from SVM only became more competitive when using features extracted from Zernike moments, while J48 performance was better in the situations where the features from Haralick moments were in the dataset. Regarding to Random Forest and MLP, they showed a progressive increase in performance as the authors changed images representation.

So, the best results overall were achieved when the authors represented the thermographic images using the combination of the features from Haralick and Zernike moments. MLP outperformed the others methods in all situations, indicating that even being a two-class problem, the detection of breast lesion in thermographic images is a complex task to be handled.

Table 6 is the confusion matrix for the best classification, which was achieved using the combination of both features descriptors and MLP classifier. The confusion matrix matches the result in Table 5, since the amount of correctly classified instances is much greater than the misclassified instances. However, the matrix also shows that there was more false negative results than false positive, which is something to be concerned in this kind of application.

CONCLUSION

This chapter assessed the performance of different intelligent methods in identifying breast lesions in thermographic images in frontal view. The authors also tested different ways to represent the images using Haralick moments and Zernike moments. From this study, they found that in this situation, the best approach was to combine the features extracted from both descriptors. The Multilayer Perceptron network outperformed the others methods, achieving up to 95% of accuracy. This result shows a sensibility of 96.92% and specificity of 93.40%.

Future studies may optimize diagnosis, reducing the amount of misclassification, especially reducing the amount of false negative results. In this way, the authors may use some other computational tools such as features selection methods, to reduce features redundancy, thus improving images representation, or other classification methods based on deep learning, in order to minimize the amount of incorrectly classified instances. The proposed method showed to be promising and, in the future, it may be used in an application for breast cancer screening.

ACKNOWLEDGMENTS

The authors thank Coordenação de Aperfeiçoamento de Pessoal de Nível Superior (CAPES), Brazil and to Fundação de Amparo à Ciência e Tecnologia de Pernambuco (FACEPE), Brazil for the support in the research.

REFERENCES

[1] Stewart, B. W., and Wild, C. P. (2014). *World Cancer Report.* Lyon: International Agency for Research on Cancer Press.

[2] Usuki, H., Tilkeda, Igarachi, Y., Takahashi, I., Fukami, A., Yokoe, T., Sonoo, H., and Asaishi, K. (1998). "What kinds of non-palpable breast cancer can be detected by thermography?" *Biomedical Thermology* 18(4): 8-12.

[3] Borchartt, T. B. (2013). *Análise de imagens termográficas para a classificação de alterações na mama [Thermographic image analysis*

for breast alteration classification] PhD diss., Fluminense Federal University, Brazil.

[4] Resmini, R., Conci, A., Borchartt, T. B., Lima, R. C. F., Montenegro, A. A., and Pantaleão, C. A. (2012). "Diagnóstico Precoce de Doenças Mamárias Usando Imagens Térmicas e Aprendizado de Máquina." ["Early Diagnosis of Breast Diseases Using Thermal Imaging and Machine Learning."] *Revista Eletrônica do Alto Vale do Itajaí* 1(1): 55-67.

[5] Hendrick, R. E. (2010). "Radiation doses and cancer risks from breast imaging studies." *Radiology* 25(1): 246-253.

[6] Freitas Júnior, R., Fiori, W. F., Ramos, F. J. F, Godinho, E., Rahal, R. M. S., and Oliveira, J. G. (2006). "Discomfort and pain during mammography." *Revista da Associação Médica Brasileira* 52(5): 333-336.

[7] Lahiri, B. B., Bagavathiappan, S., Jayakumar, T., and Philip, J. (2012). "Medical applications of infrared thermography: A review." *Infrared Physics & Technology* 55(4): 221-235.

[8] Liao, S. X., and Pawlak, M. (1998). "On the accuracy of Zernike moments for image analysis." *IEEE Transactions on Pattern Analysis and Machine Intelligence* 20(12): 1358-1364.

[9] Haralick, R. M., Shanmugam, K., and Dinstein, I. H. (1973). "Textural Features for Image Classification." *IEEE Transactions on Systems, Man, and Cybernetics* SMC-3(6): 610-621.

[10] Osareh, A., and Shadgar, B. (2010). "Machine learning techniques to diagnose brast cancer." Paper presented at *2010 5th International Symposium on Health Informatics and Bioinformatics*, Antalya, Turkey, April 20-22.

[11] Wahab, A. A., Salim, M. I., Ahamat, M. A., Manaf, N. A., Yunus, J., and Lai, K. W. (2016). "Thermal distribution analysis of three-dimensional tumor-embedded breast models with different breast density compositions." *Medical & Biological Engineering & Computing* 54(9): 1363-1373.

[12] Wakankar, A. T., and Suresh, G. R. (2016). "Automatic Diagnosis of Breast Cancer using Thermographic Color Analysis and SVM

Classifier." In: *Intelligent Systems Technologies and Applications 2016*, edited by Corchado, R. J., Mitra, S., Thampi, S., and El-Alfy, E. S., 21-32. Cham: Springer.

[13] Milosevic, M., Jankovic, D., and Peulic, A. (2014). "Thermography based breast cancer detection using texture features and minimum variance quantization." *EXCLI Journal* 13: 1204-1215.

[14] Borchartt. T. B., Conci, A., Lima, R. C., Resmini, R., and Sanchez, A. (2013). "Breast thermography from an image processing viewpoint: A survey." *Signal Processing* 93(10): 2785-2803.

[15] Cheng, H. D., Shi, X. J., Min, R., Hu, L. M., Cai, X. P., and Du, H. N. (2006). "Approaches for automated detection and classification of masses in mammograms." *Pattern Recognition* 39(4): 646-668.

[16] Azevedo, W. W., Lima, S. M. L., Fernandes, I. M. M., Rocha, A. D. D., Cordeiro, F. R., Silva-Filho, A. G., and Santos, W. P. (2015). "Morphological extreme learning machines applied to detect and classify masses in mammograms" Paper presented at *2015 International Joint Conference of Neural Networks (IJCNN)*, Killarney, Ireland

[17] Pramanik. S., Bhattacharjee, D., and Nasipuri, M. (2015). "Wavelet based thermogram analysis for breast cancer detection." Paper presented at *2015 International Symposium on Advanced Computing and Communication (ISACC)*, Silchar, India, September 14-15.

[18] Santana, M. A., Pereira, J. M. S., Silva, F. L., Lima, N. M., Sousa, F. N., Arruda, G. M. S., Lima, R. C. F., Silva, W. W. A., and Santos, W. P. (2018). "Breast cancer diagnosis based on mammary thermography and extreme learning machines." *Research on Biomedical Engineering* 34(1):45-53. Epub March 05, 2018. https://dx.doi.org/ 10.1590/2446-4740.05217.

[19] Oliveira, M. M. (2012). *Desenvolvimento de protocolo e construção de um aparato mecânico para padronização da aquisição de imagens termográficas de mama* [Protocol development and construction of a mechanical apparatus for standardization of breast thermographic imaging] PhD diss., Federal University of Pernambuco, Brazil.

[20] Silva, A. S. V. (2015). *Classificação e segmentação de termogramas de mama para triagem de pacientes residentes em regiões de poucos recursos médicos* [Classification and segmentation of breast thermograms for screening patients residing in low-resource regions] PhD diss., Federal University of Pernambuco, Brazil.

[21] Oliveira, L. F., Narloch, A. L. M., Kist, D. M., Soares Filho, M. P., Meneghello, G. E., Cavalheiro, G. G. H., and Tillmann, M. A. A. (2012). "Extração de Características de Forma utilizando matriz de co-ocorrência e Atributos de Haralick" ["Extracting Shape Characteristics Using Co-Occurrence Matrix and Haralick Attributes."] Paper presented at *2012 Workshop de Visão Computacional*, Goiânia, Brazil, May 27-30.

[22] Felipe, J. C., Olioti, J. B., and Traina, A. J. M. (2005). "Discriminação de Aspectos Malignos em Massas Tumorais de Mamografias Usando Características de Forma das Imagens" ["Discrimination of Malignant Aspects in Mammogram Tumor Masses Using Image Shape Characteristics"]. Paper presented at *V Workshop de Informática Médica*, Porto Alegre, Brazil, June.

[23] Lima, S. M. L, Silva-Filho, A. G., and Santos, W. P. (2016). "Detection and classification of masses in mammographic images in a multi-kernel approach." *Computer Methods and Programs in Biomedicine* 134:11-29. doi: 10.1016/j.cmpb.2016.04.029.

[24] Tahmasbi, A., Saki, F., and Shokouhi, S. B. (2011). "Classification of benign and malignant masses based on Zernike moments." *Computers in Biology and Medicine* 41(8): 726-735.

[25] Heckerman, D., Geiger, D., and Chickering, D. M. (1995). "Learning Bayesian Networks: The combination of knowledge and statistical data." *Machine Learning* 20(3): 197-243.

[26] Patil, T. R., and Sherekar, S. S. (2013). "Performance analysis of Naïve Bayes and J48 classification algorithm for data classification." *International Journal of Computer Science and Applications* 6(2): 256-261.

[27] Valença, M. (2010). *Fundamentos das Redes Neurais*. 2nd ed. Brazil: Livro Rápido.

[28] Platt, J. C. (1998). *Sequential Minimal Optimization: A Fast Algorithm for Training Support Vector Machines*. Technical Report MSR-TR-98-14, USA: Microsoft.
[29] Ho, T. K. (1995). "Random decision forests." Paper presented at the *3rd International Conference on Document Analysis and Recognition*, Montreal, Canada, August 14-16.
[30] Breiman, L. 2001. "Random Forests." *Machine Learning* 45(1): 5-32.
[31] Amit, Y., and Geman, D. (1996). "Shape quantization and recognition with randomized trees." *Neural Computation* 9(7): 1545-1588.
[32] Geurts, P., Ernst, D., and Wehenkel, L. (2006). "Extremely randomized trees." *Machine Learning* 63: 3-42.
[33] Quinlan, R. (1993). *Programs for machine learning*. San Francisco: Morgan Kaufmann.
[34] Hall, M., Frank, E., Holmes, G., Pfahringer, B., Reutemann, P., and Witten, I. H. (2009). "The WEKA Data Mining Software: An Update." *SIGKDD Explorations* 11(1).
[35] Jung, Y., and Hu, J. (2015). "A k-fold averaging cross-validation procedure." *Journal of Nonparametric Statistics* 27(2): 167-179.

In: Understanding a Cancer Diagnosis
Editors: W. P. dos Santos et al.
ISBN: 978-1-53617-520-2
© 2020 Nova Science Publishers, Inc.

Chapter 5

DIALECTICAL OPTIMIZATION METHOD AS A FEATURE SELECTION TOOL FOR BREAST CANCER DIAGNOSIS USING THERMOGRAPHIC IMAGES

Jessiane Mônica Silva Pereira[1],
Maíra Araújo de Santana[2],
Washington Wagner Azevedo da Silva[2],
Rita de Cássia Fernandes de Lima[3],
Sidney Marlon Lopes de Lima[4]
and Wellington Pinheiro dos Santos[2,*]

[1]Polytechnique School of the University of Pernambuco, Recife, Brazil
[2]Department of Biomedical Engineering,
[3]Department of Mechanical Engineering,
[4]Department of Electronics and Systems,
Federal University of Pernambuco, Recife, Brazil

---

* Corresponding Author's Email: wellington.santos@ufpe.br

Abstract

Cancer is a leading cause of death and has become one of the biggest public health issues in the world. Early detection and treatment are essential to minimize the effects of this disease, reducing mortality rates. In order to reduce mortality, alternatives tools for early detection of tumors appear. In this context arises the thermography applied to mastology. Breast thermography assessment is possible due to metabolic changes resulting from the presence of cancer cells in the breast tissue. These mutant cells change in the temperature distribution in the breast. Thermography has been used as a complementary technique to mammography, serving as a screening system. Since these metabolic changes appear at early stages of cancer, the use of thermography may allow early detection of breast lesions. Despite being a promising technique, the interpretation of thermographic images is often difficult. It becomes more difficult when the lesions are far from skin surface. Thus, pattern recognition techniques are being explored as an important tool to aid diagnosis. When using pattern recognition algorithms, images are represented by features vectors. Features selection plays an important role within this process. Its goal is to reduce the search space, but avoiding major changes in the accuracy of the breast lesion classification. This study aims to develop a features selection model based on the dialectical optimization algorithm (ODM) and using an Extreme Learning Machine (ELM) as the objective function. This method was applied to the features extracted from the thermographic images, to optimize breast lesions diagnosis. From the results presented in this chapter, the authors found that the combination of ODM and ELM resulted in a reduction of about 57% of the features vector. The results also reduced the average accuracy in around 6% to 10%. Thus, they found that ODM combined to ELM is a promising method for features selection. Further tests may be performed, not only to find the smallest dimension of the features vector, but also reduce the impact in classification accuracy.

Keywords: breast cancer, thermography, features selection, optimization and classification

Introduction

Cancer is a leading cause of death and has become one of the biggest public health issues in the world. For decades, breast cancer has been the most common type of cancer among women. It is currently ranked among the top five causes of cancer death worldwide (WHO, 2018). Early detection has been proven to be the key tool to minimize the effects of this disease. The sooner the disease is detected, the more successful the treatment can be, thus, reducing mortality rates [1].

Nowadays, some imaging techniques are used to detect breast cancer. The most common techniques are mammography, ultrasonography, magnetic resonance imaging, x-ray tomography and thermography. The combination of these techniques is also assessed to provide a robust and more accurate diagnosis. Among these screening tools, mammography is the most widely used. It is a low-dose x-ray procedure and is considered the gold standard for breast cancer diagnosis. Yet, mammography has some limitations. Among its main limitations are the cost of the exam and the exposure to cumulative ionizing radiation, which is a risk factor for cancer. Another important concern is the high false negative rates among young women, since their breasts tend to have mostly dense tissue, which appear on the same color of a lesion in mammographic image [1].

Thermography is being used as an auxiliary screening tool for breast cancer. In this technique, the image is acquired by an infrared camera. The camera captures infrared radiation emitted by the surface of interest. The resulting image shows the surface temperature distribution. Therefore, there is no need for invasive procedures or exposure to ionizing radiation. In addition, this technique provides physiological information, since damaged areas show increased metabolic activity. More cellular activity increases the temperature around the area, so breast lesions can be seen as warmer spots. Considering that physiological alterations precede anatomical alterations, the use of this technique is a great step for early diagnosis [2].

Despite being a promising technique, the interpretation of thermographic images is often difficult. It becomes more difficult when the lesions are far from the surface of the skin. In these cases, changes in temperature occur in a diffuse and non-punctual manner. Thus, pattern recognition techniques are being explored as an important tool to support diagnosis.

When using pattern recognition algorithms, images are represented by feature vectors. In the approach presented in this chapter, the authors chose to use Haralick moments and Zernike moments as features extractors. Zernike moments extract geometry information, while Haralick is associated to texture characteristics.

Another important step in optimizing the performance of intelligent systems is the features selection. This step plays a key role in reducing computational costs and increasing accuracy as it seeks to remove irrelevant and redundant features. In this study, the authors propose a feature selection approach combining the Dialectical Optimization Method (ODM) and Extreme Learning Machines (ELM).

The optimization and search methods present in literature are mostly inspired by nature. This inspiration may be seen in Genetic Algorithms (GA), in the bee colony-based algorithm and in the Particle Swarm Optimization (PSO) methods. The Dialectical Optimization Method (ODM) is an evolution and revolution based tool to perform search and optimization tasks [3].

Given this, this study proposes to model the features selection method based on the dialectical method of optimization. The authors chose to use ELM classifier as the objective function of the ODM. ELM is a learning technique proposed for training feedfoward neural networks with a single hidden layer that accelerates learning by randomly generating random weights for both input and hidden layers [4].

In the first section of this chapter, the methods section, the authors present the basic concepts and definition, the proposed method, a description of the database and the tools used to perform the tests. In the results and discussion section, they present the results from the experiments and perform some qualitative and quantitative analyzes from them. Finally, they summarize the scientific contribution of this approach and discuss the potential future studies.

METHODS

Breast Thermography

Breast cancer is one of the most common types of cancer among women, and still represents the highest mortality rate from cancer. In an attempt to reduce mortality, health professionals are investing on alternative tools to provide an early detection of lesions, improving prognosis. The most used methods, such as mammography, ultrasound, magnetic resonance imaging and clinical examination, are proving to be less effective in detecting early stages of breast lesions. This happens since younger women have breasts with higher density tissues, making it difficult to identify and differentiate the lesions from the images [5].

Thermography has become an auxiliary tool in the process of diagnosing breast cancer. This technique uses an infrared camera to acquire images that present the temperature distribution in the region. The camera captures the infrared radiation emitted by the surface of interest. It is a non-invasive process where the patient is not exposed to any ionizing radiation. This technique access metabolic changes resulting from the appearance of altered cells in the breast tissue. Cancer cells increased activity leads to changes in temperature distribution in the breast surface [6].

Features Selection

For machine learning field, an important step is the features selection. This step aims to rank the features according to some criteria of importance. So, it is possible to reduce the dimensionality of the features search space and remove noisy data. Thus, features selection may be seen as a search process where an algorithm must find the smallest subset of features that result in the best classification performance [7].

There are basically two different approaches to handle features selection: Wrapper and Filter. The first approach deals essentially with the use of the classifier system itself as a metric to check the performance of many features subsets. In the second approach, heuristic metrics are used to try to find a subset that meets some criterion or metrics [8]. The features selection method used in this paper will be detailed in the following section.

Dialectical Optimization Method

Dialectical Optimization Method (ODM) is a class of evolutionary algorithm to be adapted to search and optimization problems. It is based on the concepts of evolution and revolution. [9, 10].

The origin of the word "dialectic" comes from the original Greek dialetiké. The prefix "dia" corresponds to interaction, while "letiké" stands for knowledge. Thus, for Socratic philosophers, dialectics are seen as "the art of dialogue". In this way, dialectics is seen as the free interaction between contrary ideas about an object, and it is possible to obtain information about the truth of an object. [11].

The dialectical method and its modern definition began in the late 18th and early 19th centuries through the works of the German philosopher George Wilhelm Friedrich Hegel, 1770-1831. This definition was developed with influence on the Eastern dialectical conceptions brought from China by the Jesuits and on the Heraclitus' thinking of reality as a process of eternal modification [10].

The ODM is based on the conception of parts of reality, or phenomena, as systems. The systems consist of several poles. Each pole has a force or power. The system is then characterized by its correlation of forces, that is, by the grouping of the forces of its component poles. This interaction follows the model conceived by Hegel and based on three fundamental concepts. The first concept is the contradiction, which is the basis of dialectic and is defined by the correlation between the forces of the poles over time. The second concept is the principle of totality, which defines that a totally isolated system cannot be conceived, but in its various relations and dependencies with other systems. The third is the endless movement, which, as the name implies, expresses the fundamental dialectic hypothesis that there is nothing eternal, nothing fixed, nothing absolute. In this way, the dialectic and the movement of contradictions [12].

The dialectical method adapted to search and optimization problems considers each pole as a possible candidate for the problem. Thus, it is necessary to associate the objective function of the optimization problem to the social force of each pole. So the dynamics of the optimization method is governed by the poles fight. These struggles consist of the movement of the poles, which happens due to the present hegemonic pole and the historical hegemonic pole. The present hegemonic pole is the one with the largest social force in the current correlation of forces, whereas the historical hegemonic pole is the one with the greatest historical force to date [12].

The search for possible solutions is intrinsically associated with the pole movement and its contradictions in the various historical phases, which are involved in periods of revolutionary crisis. In this period occurs the fusion of poles with low levels of contradiction, the creation of new poles by synthesis in order to solve high levels of contradiction and also the formation of absolute antithesis of the poles thesis. Still, at this stage, there is a process to generate diversity in the search process that corresponds to adding disturbances to the surviving poles, which is a process similar to mutation in evolutionary-based computational approaches [12].

To understand the objective dialectical method for search and optimization, it is necessary to understand the following general definition.

General Definition
The basic concepts of dialectics were mathematically defined as follows [9]:

Pole
It is a candidate for the solution of the problem and also the fundamental unit of the dialectical system. Given a set of poles $\Omega = \{w_1, w_2, ..., w_m\}$ one pole w_i is associated to a weight vector $w_i = (w_{i,1}, w_{i,2}, ..., w_{i,n})_T$ where $w_i \in s$, m is the number of poles and n is the dimensionality of the system.

Social Force

Evaluation through the objective function for a pole. Each pole w_i has a social force that equals the evaluation of the objective function f at pole w_i.

Hegemony

In the process of pole fighting, it is said that a pole k exerts hegemony at time t if:

$$f(w_k(t)) = f_C(t) = \max f(w_j(t)), 1 \leq j \leq m(t)$$

The vector $w_C(t) = w_k(t)$ is called present hegemonic pole or contemporary hegemonic pole, while $f_C(t)$ is the present hegemonic force or contemporary hegemonic force. The historical hegemonic force at the instant t, $f_H(t)$ is expressed by:

$$f_H(t) = \max f_C(t'), \text{onde } w_H = w_H, \text{para } f(w_C(t')) = f_H(t) e\ 0 \leq t' \leq t$$

Absolute Antithesis

The absolute antithesis vector of the pole w is defined as the opposite vector to w and can be expressed as: $w = s_i - x_i + r_i$, where $i = 1, 2, \cdots, n$. Thus assuming $x = (x_1, x_2, \ldots x_n)^T$ and that $x \in s \Rightarrow r_i \leq x_i \leq s_i$, and r_i and s_i correspond to the lower and upper limits of the i-th dimension of, s.

Contradiction

Contradiction can be calculated from a distance function, which in this case is the Euclidean distance. Thus we can mathematically define the distance between two poles w_p and w_q through:

$$\delta_{p,q} = d(w_p, w_q)$$

Synthesis

Based on the dialectical conception, synthesis is the answer to the contradiction between two poles where one plays the role of thesis and the other of antithesis. Given a pole $w_r \in s$ whose synthesis between poles w_p and w_q can be obtained through the expression: $w_r = g(w_p, w_t)$, where $g: S^2 \to S$ there are possible synthesis days:

$$w_{u,i} = \begin{cases} w_{p,i}, & i \bmod 2 = 0 \\ w_{q,i}, & i \bmod 2 = 1 \end{cases}, i = 1, 2, \ldots, n$$

$$w_{u,i} = \begin{cases} w_{p,i}, & i \bmod 2 = 1 \\ w_{q,i}, & i \bmod 2 = 0 \end{cases}, i = 1, 2, \ldots, n$$

Based on these definitions it is possible to build the dialectical method as the search and optimization algorithm that will be shown in the following section.

Dialectic Method as Search and Optimization Algorithm

To use the dialectical method in a search and optimization problem (such as features selection), it is necessary to understand the adaptation that is shown below and proposed by Santos and Assis (2013) [12].

First of all, we define the fundamental parameters, which are the initial number of poles, $m(0)$, number of historical phases n_p and duration of each historical phase n_H. Thus, the system will be started with $m(0)$ poles and will last n_p historical phases with n_H generations per phase. The number of poles $m(0)$ corresponds to the concept of initial population when compared to evolutionary approaches, it must be even so that half of the poles are randomly generated and the other half is obtained by generating the absolute antithesis poles. This process generates a more intense pole fight, generating a greater initial dynamic.

The phase of poles generation is performed according to the following expression:

$$w_{i,j}(0) = \begin{cases} U(r_j, s_j), & 1 \leq i \leq m(0) \\ w_{i',j}(0), & 1 + \frac{1}{2}m(0) \leq i \leq m(0) \end{cases}$$

$$w_{i',j} = s_j - w_{i,j} + r_j$$

For $i' = 1 + \frac{1}{2}m(0) \leq i \leq m(0)$, $1 \leq i \leq m(0)$ and $1 \leq j \leq n$, where n is the dimensionality of the optimization problem, $U(r_j, s_j)$ is a random number evenly distributed over the range $[r_j, s_j]$ and $S = [r_1, s_1] \times [r_2, s_2] \times ... \times [r_n, s_n]$, since $s_j > r_j$ and $s_j, r_j \in \mathbb{R}$.

While it does not reach the number of historical phases n_p and the historical hegemonic force is not higher than the given upper force threshold (initial estimate of the maximum objective function value), $f_H(t) < f_{sup}$ (criterion to consider the maximum objective function achieved), there is the stage of evolution and revolutionary crisis. Evolution occurs until the total of n_H iterations and $f_H(t) < f_{sup}$ is reached, thus the poles are adjusted as follows.

$$w_i(t+1) = w_i(t) + \Delta w_{C,i}(t) + \Delta w_{H,i}(t),$$

to

$$\Delta w_{C,i} = \eta_{C,i}(t)\left(1 - \mu_C(t)\right)^2 \left(w_C(t) - w_i(t)\right), 0 < \eta_C(t), 1,$$
$$\Delta w_{H,i} = \eta_{H,i}(t)\left(1 - \mu_H(t)\right)^2 \left(w_H(t) - w_i(t)\right), 0 < \eta_H(t), 1,$$

where $\eta_C(0) = \eta_H(0) = \eta_0$ and $0 < \eta_0 < 1$. The influences of present and historical hegemonies are modeled by the following terms $\Delta w_{C,i}(t)$ and $\Delta w_{H,i}(t)$, respectively, on the i-th pole. The present and historical poles update step are represented by $\eta_C(t)$ and $\eta_H(t)$. This update occurs at each historical phase as defined in the expression below.

$$\eta_C(t+1) = \alpha\, \eta_C(t)$$

And for every interaction occurs:

$$\eta_H(t+1) = \alpha\, \eta_H(t)$$

At the end of each historical phase, to $\alpha < 1$ (typically, $\alpha = 0{,}9999$). The present pertinence degree and the historical relevance degree correspond to the terms $\mu_{C,i}(t)$ and $\mu_{H,i}(t)$, these terms are based on the pertinence functions according to the expressions described below.

$$\mu_{C,i}(t) = \sum_{j=1}^{m} \left(\frac{|f(w_i(t)) - f_C(t)|}{|f(w_j(t)) - f_C(t)|}\right)^{-1}, \text{ where } 1 < i < m(t)$$

$$\mu_{H,i}(t) = \sum_{j=1}^{m} \left(\frac{|f(w_i(t)) - f_H(t)|}{|f(w_j(t)) - f_H(t)|}\right)^{-1}, \text{ where } 1 < i < m(t)$$

Where these expressions are based on the membership functions of the classical version of the unsupervised fuzzy c-average classifier proposed by Zhu and Jiang (2003) [27]. Thus, when the social force of the i-th pole, $f(w_i(t))$ is close to the present hegemonic force $f_C(t)$, the term of $\mu_{C,i}(t)$ is close to 1 making the influence of present hegemony $\Delta w_{C,i}(t)$ approaches zero and practically student its effect and similar behavior happens when $f(w_i(t))$ approaches the value of historical hegemonic force $f_H(t)$.

In the revolutionary crisis stage all contradictions are evaluated and contradictions smaller than a minimal contradiction (δmin) imply fusion between the poles. From the contradictions evaluated in the previous step, those greater than one maximum contradiction (δmax) are found. These contradictions will be considered the main contradictions of the dialectic system. The thesis-antithesis pairs are involved, whose synthesis poles also pass to belong to the new set of poles.

Additionally there is the effect of the crisis given by the maximum crisis ($Xmax$), to all poles belonging to the dialectic system, thus generating a new set of poles, according to the following expression.

$$w_{k,i}(t+2) = w_{k,i}(t+1) + Xmax\, G(0,1),$$

To $1 \leq k \leq m(t+1)$ and $1 \leq i \leq n$, where $G(0,1)$ is a random number from a gaussian distribution with hope 0 and variance 1.

If the stopping criterion has not yet been met (maximum number of historical phases reached or another stopping criterion to be defined), a new set of poles is generated. This is a step called antagonistic poles generation that is given by the expression below:

$$w_i(t+2) \in \Omega(t+2) \Rightarrow w\ (t+2) + \in \Omega(t+2),$$

to $1 \leq i \leq m(t+2)$, where $m(t+2) = 2m(t+1)$.

In this way it is possible to enlarge the set of poles by adding the antithetical poles to the existing poles.

Figure 1 shows the general fluxogram of the dialectical optimization method adapted for search and optimization tasks. In summary, it can be stated that the pole evolution phase is composed of the hegemony search and weight update stages that model the iterations between the poles and the information exchange over time. While the crisis phase is composed of the stages of evaluation, fusion, synthesis, revolutionary crisis and generation of antithesis pairs. It is also understood that the stage of synthesis occurs the separation of groups of poles that are between two ideological extremes during the crisis, while the generation stage of the antagonistic poles models the emergence of groups with ideas totally contrary to those of the current group. The fusion stage of low contradictions shapes the union of poles that have similar thinking in times of crisis [13].

In this study, the objective function, which calculates the social force of each pole of this method, was applied a classifier in order to minimize the error rate in the classification process. The classifier used was Extreme Learning Machine (ELM), which is a training approach for single hidden layer Neural Networks.

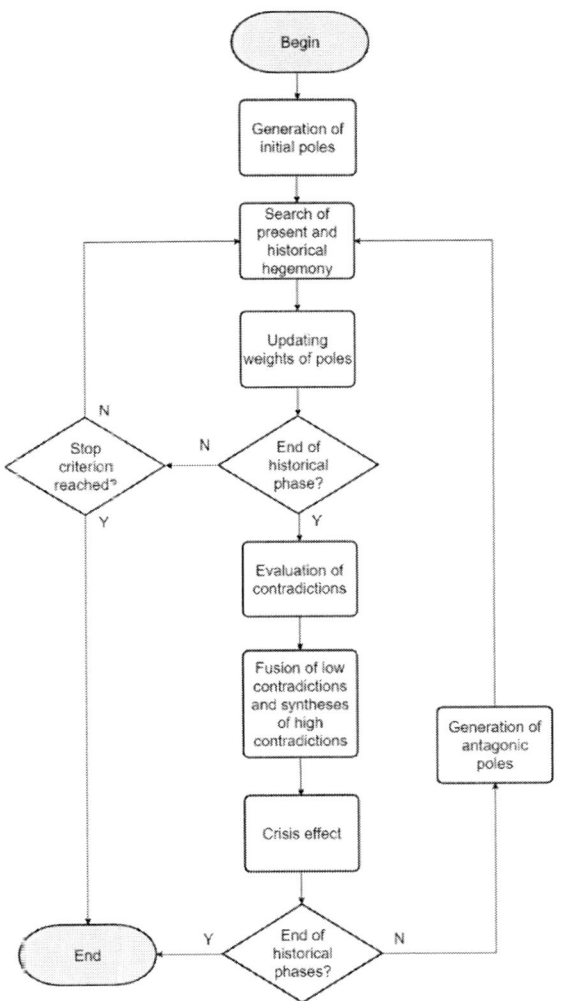

Source: Adapted from [12].

Figure 1. General flow chart of the dialectical optimization method adapted to search and optimization tasks.

Extreme Learning Machines

Artificial Neural Networks (RNA) are computational techniques that present a mathematical model inspired by the structure of a neuron. These networks are composed of neurons, interacting through synapses, just like biological neurons. Neural networks modify their synaptic weights to achieve desired outputs and, therefore, have the ability to learn and generalize. So they can generate appropriate results for conditions or situations that were not present in the learning phase and can solve many complex problems [4].

The ELM is a training approach for single middle layer Neural Networks. This learning technique was proposed for training single-layer feedfoward neural networks that accelerates learning by randomly generating weights from both input and hidden layers [4].

Proposed Method

This section presents the method from this approach, highlighting how the study will be conducted, as shown in Figure 2. The steps will be further described below.

The thermographic images used in this study follow the acquisition protocol proposed in Oliveira (2012) [14] and were acquired at Hospital das Clínicas (HC) - UFPE. According to Silva (2015) [15] the thermographic images were obtained from a FLIR S45 infrared camera and the method adopted in the image acquisition process was the static one, in the static acquisition the patient is in thermal equilibrium with the environment. Eight (8) images were obtained from each patient in JPG format, each image being named: T1 (frontal with hands on waist), T2 (frontal with hands raised holding a bar above the head), internal side of breast right breast (LIMD), left breast internal lateral (LIME), right breast external lateral (LEMD) and left breast external lateral (LEME). Example of the eight images obtained from each patient can be seen in Figure 3. In this chapter, only frontal images T1 and T2 were used, as this condition is considered to benefit the identification of the region of interest.

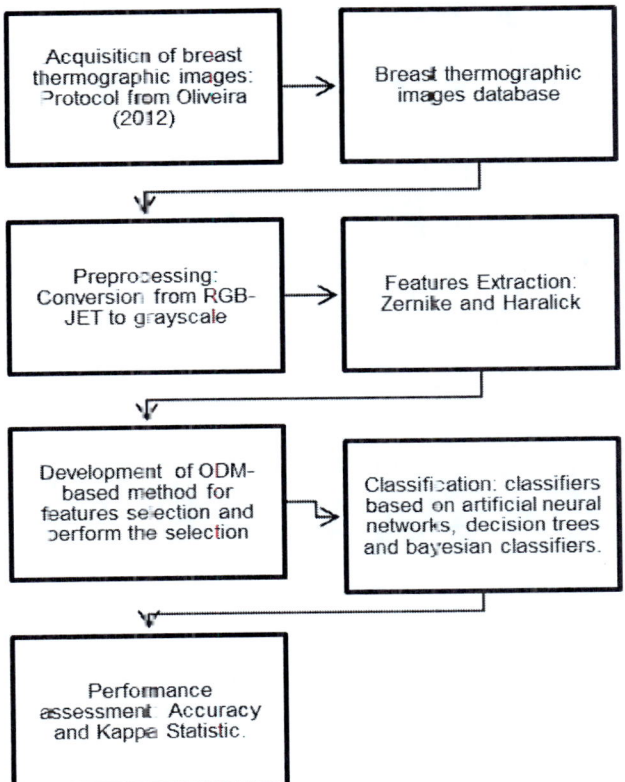

Source: The authors.

Figure 2. General flow chart of the dialectical optimization method adapted to search and optimization tasks.

The database has been labeled using established diagnostic methods as described by Dourado Neto (2014) [16]. The database is separated into four classes: Malignant Lesion, Benign Lesion, Cyst and No Lesion. The Malignant Lesion class comprises all cases of biopsy-proven malignant breast injury. The Benign Lesion class refers to cases of tumors with benignity, also confirmed by biopsy. The Cyst class includes cases with this diagnosis proven by fine needle aspiration (FNA) or ultrasound [15]. The No Lesion class is composed of all images that did not present an injury.

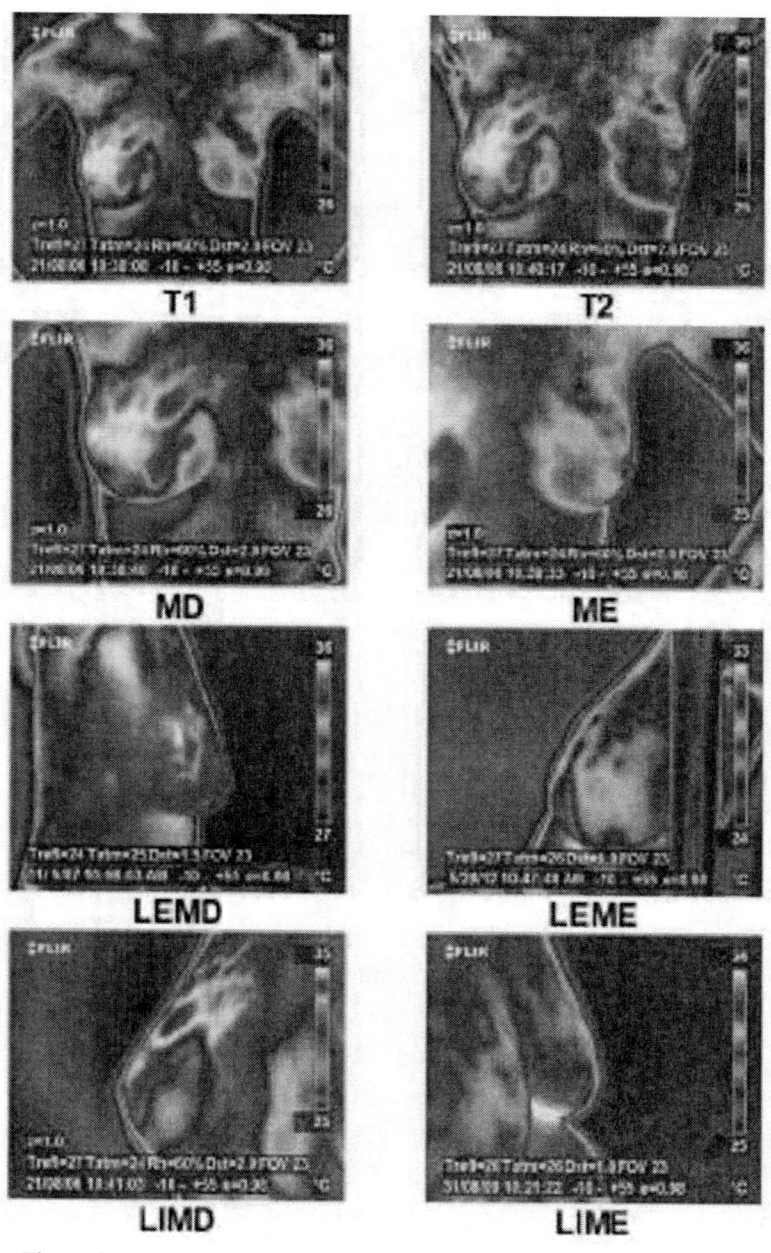

Source: The authors.

Figure 3. Positions for the eight images acquired from each patient.

Thermographic images use pseudo-coloring techniques. For this database, the JET color palette was used in the acquisition process. Therefore, it was necessary to use the conversion from RGB-JET to grayscale, in order to reduce the amount of information to be processed. Grayscale images have less detail but retain the important features of objects or regions of interest [17].

The definition of the feature extraction method is one of the most important factors for the satisfactory performance of a computer system for diagnosis support [18].

Regarding to image representation, the features in this chapter were based on geometry or texture. The authors used the Zernike moments features extractor, that extracts geometry-based information and the Haralick moments extractor, which is based on texture features. The first one is from projections of the image function on orthogonal base functions and only rotation invariants [19]. The second calculates texture information from the co-occurrence matrix of the image, which quantifies some characteristics from gray level variation of these images [18, 19]. Thus, the extracted features were organized in an ARFF format file, in which a total of 168 attributes and 968 instances were counted.

The number of images per class in the database is different, which may lead to biased result during training, in a way that injuries could be more often classified in the class that has the largest number of instances. In order to solve this problem, the authors performed a class balancing by inserting synthetic instances through the linear combination of features vectors of the same class [20].

As stated earlier, the dialectical method can be used in a search and optimization problem, such as features selection. Features selection plays an essential role within machine learning process. Its goal is to reduce the computational cost of the system, but always taking into account the need to maintain high performance rates during the classification [7].

When using ODM for features selection, the poles were represented by numerical vectors containing their binary values dimensions using a threshold of (0.5). In the dialectical method, as already described, half of the poles are created with random values and the other half is generated by the poles that are antagonistic to the first half of poles already initialized. The aptitude values are obtained by defining the objective function, which in this case will be the minimum error rate of the ELM classifier. This error in this technique is known as social force.

The parameters used for this approach were obtained by successive executions of the algorithm, changing the parameters and, thus, saving the parameter values from where the authors found the lowest error rate at the end of each execution. Table 1 shows the ODM parameters for the lowest error rate in this study.

Table 1. Parameters used for ODM

Initial number of poles	10
Pole Dimension	168
Number of Historical Phases	1
Duration of each Historic Phase	500
Superior Range	1
Inferior Range	0
Alpha	0,999
Eta L	0,999
Eta H	1,001
Maximum Contradiction	0,0005
Minimal Contradiction	0,001
Maximum Crisis Effect	0,005

The authors performed classification before and after the features selection step to assess the efficiency of the feature selection process. Thus, these features are used as input for classifiers who will be trained and will later perform classification of breast lesions (malignant, benign and cyst) or no lesion. This experiment was performed with seven classifiers to compare their ability to detect and classify breast lesions in thermographic images. The classifiers used were: Bayes Net, Naive Bayes, SVM, J48, MLP, Random Forest and Random Tree.

Naive Bayes and Bayes Net are Bayes theory-based classifiers that use conditional probability to create a data model. Bayes Net builds a complete Bayesian network and then searches that network according to any search algorithm and its main parameter is the type of search performed. Naive Bayes assumes that all features are independent, given the class variable so it is considered naive [21].

The support vector machine (SVM) classifier performs a nonlinear mapping of the dataset in a larger dimension space, and then a hyperplane is created to separate the distinct classes. SVM is based on the Statistical Learning Theory [22].

J48 classifier configures itself by creating a decision tree from a database for gaining knowledge, and thereby creating a decision-making tool. This method has the goal to build a decision tree where the most significant feature is called the root of the tree [23].

The Multilayer Perceptron (MLP) consists of a tightly connected network with feedforward connections. This neural network is a perceptron type that has a set of sensory units that make up the input layer, an intermediate or hidden layer. Its output layer consists of a layer of neurons that generate the network output. Learning in this type of network is usually performed through the backpropagation algorithm [22].

The Random Forests (RF) are decision tree combinations that hierarchically splits the data. In this method, after a certain number of trees are generated, each one casts a vote for a problem class, considering an input vector. Then, the most voted class will be chosen in the prediction of the classifier [24]. The Random Tree classifier is a decision tree that considers only a few randomly selected features for each tree node [25].

For all classifiers the training step was performed with 75% of the database and the remaining was used for test. Bayes Net, Naive Bayes, SVM, J48, MLP, Random Forest, Random Tree were also tested for the k-fold cross-validation method, with k equal to 10.

Finally, the authors assessed the different classifiers performances through the accuracy and kappa statistic. Accuracy is a percentage of correctly classified data [26]. Kappa statistic is a statistical method to evaluate the level of agreement or reproducibility of classification; it can vary between -1 and 1.

Materials

The authors used GNU/Octave, an open source environment that uses MATLAB programming language. The classification step was performed with the Waikato Environment for Knowledge Analysis (Weka) tool, version 3.8, also available for free.

RESULTS AND DISCUSSION

Both percentage split and cross-validation test methods were used for the classification in Weka. Initially, classification results were obtained using the dataset with 168 features extracted using the combination of Haralick and Zernike moments. Accuracy and Kappa statistic values can be seen in Table 2 and Table 3.

Table 2. Classification performances using all features and percentage split with 75% of database for training

	Bayes Net	Naive Bayes	MLP	SVM	J48	Random Tree	Random Forest
Accuracy	50.87	48.59	80.11	73.14	54.09	48.12	67.35
Kappa statistic	0.38	0.35	0.79	0.69	0.43	0.34	0.61

Table 3. Classification performances using all features and cross-validation with 10 folds for training

	Bayes Net	Naive Bayes	MLP	SVM	J48	Random Tree	Random Forest
Accuracy	52.61	51.63	85.79	78.65	57.88	50.97	71.28
Kappa statistic	0.37	0.35	0.81	0.71	0.44	0.34	0.61

Table 4. Classification performances after features selection using percentage split with 75% of database for training

	Bayes Net	Naive Bayes	MLP	SVM	J48	Random Tree	Random Forest
Accuracy	48.74	47.60	73.86	63.32	52.96	46.98	66.00
Kappa statistic	0.35	0.33	0.70	0.56	0.44	0.32	0.59

For the feature selection step using ODM combined to ELM method, as previously mentioned, the parameters were empirically defined, but the minimum and maximum values to be used were based on the literature. The classification results for the dataset built after the features selection are shown in Tables 4 and 5.

Table 5. Classification performances after features selection using cross-validation with 10 folds for training

	Bayes Net	Naive Bayes	MLP	SVM	J48	Random Tree	Random Forest
Accuracy	50.64	49.98	78.72	67.39	56.25	50.81	70.15
Kappa statistic	0.34	0.33	0.71	0.56	0.42	0.34	0.60

Analyzing using only the values from accuracy and kappa statistic, it is clear that the Bayesian and tree-based networks did not result in significant reductions in performance. There is a hypothesis that the evaluation function has influence on the proposed method, since ELM is inspired by neural networks.

Compared to the accuracy and kappa statistic values using neural network-based classifiers, these classifiers had a reduction of around 6% to 10% considering all results.

Regarding to the reduction of the features vector, the original vector consisted of 168 features. The number of features decreased for a vector of 72 features after the feature selection step, representing a 57% reduction in the quantity of features.

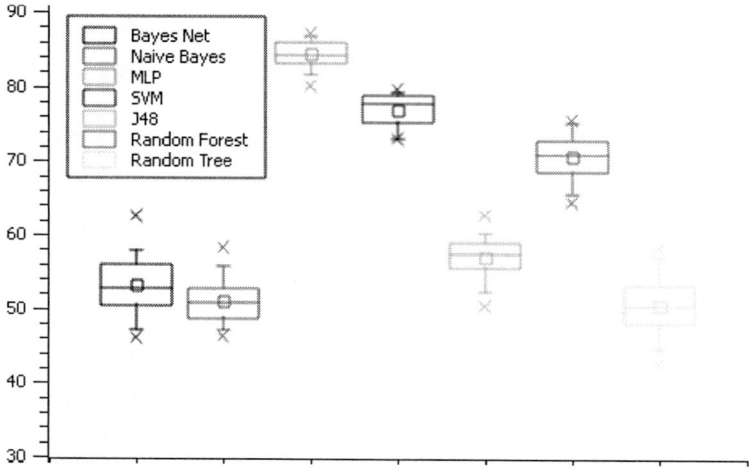

Source: The authors.

Figure 4. Boxplot for classification performances using all features and 75% of database for training.

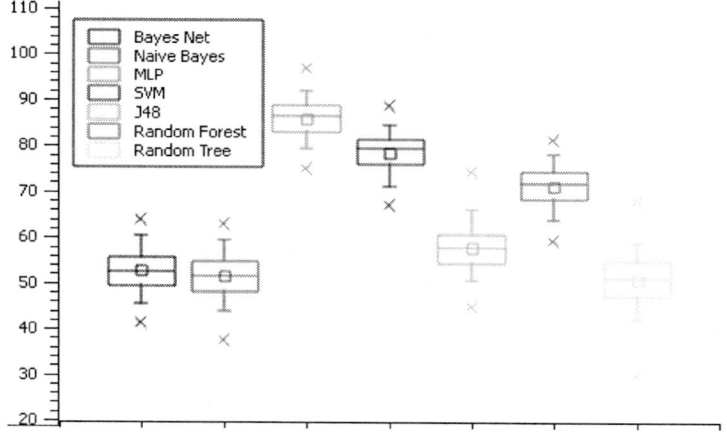

Source: The authors.

Figure 5. Boxplot for classification performances using all features and cross-validation (10 folds) for training.

To assess accuracy variation with the different classifiers, bloxplots graphs were generated to evaluate the data distribution. Figures 4 and 5 show the boxplots of all-features using the 75% training method and cross-validation method, while Figures 6 and 7 shows the results for the dataset with selected features in the same test conditions

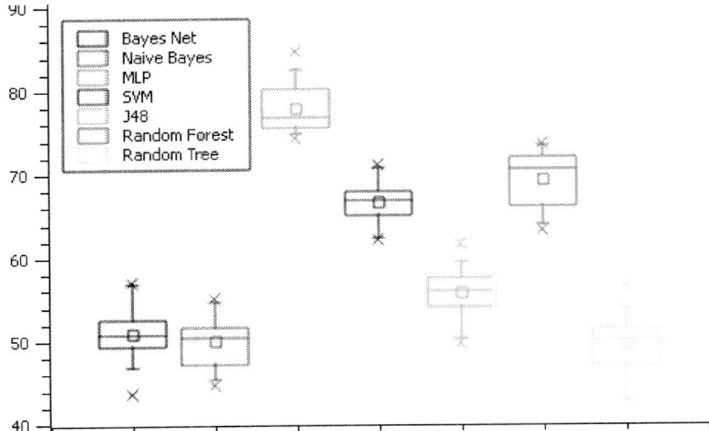

Source: The authors.

Figure 6. Boxplot for classification performances using selected features and 75% of database for training.

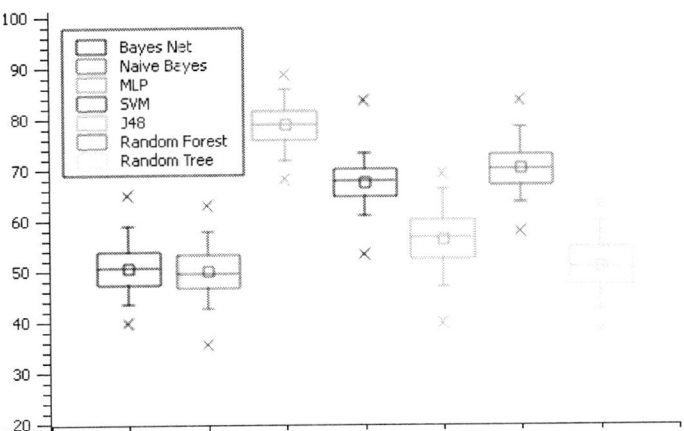

Source: The authors.

Figure 7. Boxplot for classification performances using selected features and cross-validation (10 folds) for training.

From the bloxplots, for classification accuracy before and after features selection, it is observed that there were almost no changes in the classification variability. Thus, the authors found that the feature selection method proposed in this paper does not directly affect the variability of the classification step.

Conclusion

In this study, it can be concluded that breast thermography is a good technique as a tool to help on the diagnosis of breast cancer. It is a simple technique, easy to apply and low cost that presents competitive results regarding the classification and detection of breast lesion.

This chapter proposes an approach based on ODM and ELM to reduce the number of features used to represent thermographic images from the breasts in frontal view, and thus optimize the task of classifying breast lesions. The results showed that the approach was positive, since the authors were able to significantly reduce the number of features, without considerable decrease in classification performance, when compared to the dataset using all features. However, future tests should attempt to improve classification performance, since it is a health application.

As future studies, the authors plan to explore approaches for comparing the proposed technique to more established features selection algorithms, such as genetic algorithms and particle swarm optimization. New tests should also be performed not only to find a lowest dimensionality of the features vector, but also to find a balance between the number of features and classification performance.

In order to validate the hypothesis presented in this chapter, it is necessary to change the evaluation function of the proposed methods and to observe if it has more or less influence on a classifier architecture type. Thus, the authors intend to perform tests using the tree-based classifier C4.5 and the classifier KNN as evaluation function.

ACKNOWLEDGMENTS

The authors thank the Brazilian founding agencies CAPES, CNPq and FACEPE for the partial financial support for this research.

REFERENCES

[1] American Cancer Society. (2019). *Cancer Facts & Figures*. Atlanta, GA: American Cancer Society.
[2] Etehadtavakol, M., and Ng, E. Y. K. (2013). "Breast Thermography as a Potential Non-contact Method in the Early Detection of Cancer: A review." *Journal of Mechanics in Medicine and Biology* 13(2):1330001. doi: 10.1142/S0219519413300019.
[3] Santos, W. P., and Assis, F. M. (2009). "Método Dialético de Otimização usando o Princípio da Máxima Entropia" ["Dialectical Method of Optimization using the Principle of Maximum Entropy"] *Learning and Nonlinear Models* 7(2): 54-64.
[4] Huang, G. B., Zhu, Q. Y., and Siew C. K. (2006). "Extreme learning machine: Theory and applications." *Neurocomputing* 70(1): 489–501. ISSN 09252312.
[5] Santana, M. A., Pereira, J. M. S., Silva, F. L., Lima, N. M., Sousa, F. N., Arruda, G. M. S., Lima, R. C. F., Silva, W. W. A., and Santos, W. P. (2018). "Breast cancer diagnosis based on mammary thermography and extreme learning machines." *Research on Biomedical Engineering* 34(1):45-53. Epub March 05, 2018. https://dx.doi.org/10.1590/2446-4740.05217.
[6] Silva, A. L. R. (2019). "*Seleção de atributos para apoio ao diagnóstico do câncer de mama usando imagens termográficas, algoritmos genéticos e otimização por enxame de partículas.*" ["*Selection of attributes to support breast cancer diagnosis using thermographic imaging, genetic algorithms and particle swarm*

optimization."]. Master's thesis, Federal University of Pernambuco, Brazil.

[7] Pappa, G. L., Freitas, A. A., and Kaestner, C. A. A. (2002). "A Multiobjective Genetic Algorithm for Attribute Selection." In *Proceedings of the 4th International Conference on Recent Advances in Soft Computing (RASC-2002)*, edited by Garibaldi, J., Lofti, A., and John, R., 116-121. Nottingham Trent University.

[8] Rocha, A. D. D. (2016). *"Detecção e classificação de lesões em imagens de mamografia usando classificadores SVM, wavelets morfológicas e seleção de atributos."* [*"Detection and classification of lesions in mammography images using SVM classifiers, morphological wavelets and attribute selection."*]. Master's thesis, Federal University of Pernambuco, Brazil.

[9] Santos, W. P., Souza, R. E., Santos Filho, P. B., Neto, F. B. L., and Assis, F. M. (2008). "A Dialectical Approach for Classification of DW-MR Alzheimer's Images." Paper presented at *2008 IEEE Congress on Evolutionary Computation* (IEEE World Congress on Computational Intelligence), Hong Kong, June 1-6.

[10] Santos, W. P. (2009). *"Método Dialético de Busca e Otimização para Análise de Imagens de Ressonância Magnética"* [*"Dialectical Search and Optimization Method for Magnetic Resonance Image Analysis."*] PhD diss., Federal University of Campina Grande.

[11] Vazquez, A. S. (2007). *Filosofia da Práxis*. São Paulo, Brazil: Expressão Popular [*Philosophy of Praxis*. Sao Paulo, Brazil: Popular Expression].

[12] Santos, W. P., and Assis, F. M. (2013). *Algoritmos dialéticos para inteligência computacional* [*Dialectical algorithms for computational intelligence*]. Recife, Brazil: Editora Universitária da UFPE.

[13] Feitosa, A. R. S. (2015). *"Reconstrução de imagens de tomografia por impedância elétrica utilizando o método Dialético de otimização"* [*"Reconstruction of electrical impedance tomography images using the Dialectic method of optimization."*]. Master's thesis, Federal University of Pernambuco.

[14] Oliveira, M. M. (2012). *"Desenvolvimento de protocolo e construção de um aparato mecânico para padronização da aquisição de imagens termográficas de mama."* [*"Protocol development and construction of a mechanical apparatus for standardization of breast thermographic imaging."*] Master's thesis, Federal University of Pernambuco.

[15] Silva, A. S. V. (2015). *"Classificação e segmentação de termogramas de mama para triagem de pacientes residentes em regiões de poucos recursos médicos"* [*"Classification and segmentation of breast thermograms for screening patients residing in low-resource regions"*] Master's thesis, Federal University of Pernambuco, Brazil.

[16] Dourado Neto, H. M. (2014). *"Segmentação e análise automática de termogramas: um método auxiliar na detecção do câncer de mama"* [*"Segmentation and automatic thermogram analysis: an auxiliary method for breast cancer detection"*] Master's thesis, Federal University of Pernambuco.

[17] Pedrini, H., and Schwartz, W. R. (2008). *Análise de Imagens Digitais: Princípios, Algoritmos e aplicações* [*Digital Image Analysis: Principles, Algorithms and Applications*]. São Paulo, Brazil: Thomson Learning.

[18] Cheng, H. D., Shi, X. J., Min, R., Hu, L. M., Cai, X. P., and Du, H. N. (2006). "Approaches for automated detection and classification of masses in mammograms." *Pattern Recognition* 39(4): 646-668.

[19] Shanthu, S., Bhaskaran, A. V. (2013). "A Novel Approach for detecting and Classifying Breast Cancer." *International Journal of Intelligent Information Technologies (IJIIT)* 9(1): 21-39.

[20] Lima, S. M. L, Silva-Filho, A. G., and Santos, W. P. (2016). "Detection and classification of masses in mammographic images in a multi-kernel approach." *Computer Methods and Programs in Biomedicine* 134:11-29. doi: 10.1016/j.cmpb.2016.04.029.

[21] Cheng, J., and Greiner, R. (2001). "Learning Bayesian Belief Network Classifiers: Algorithms and System." In *Proceedings of 14th Biennial Conference of the Canadian Society for Computacional Studies of Intelligence,* 141-151, Ottawa, Canada, June 7-9.

[22] Haykin, S. (1999). *Redes Neurais, Princípios e prática.* [*Neural Networks, Principles and Practice.* 2nd ed. [S.I.]: Bookman.]
[23] Librelotto, S. R. (2014). *"Análise dos algoritmos de mineração J48 e apriori aplicados na detecção de indicadores da qualidade de vida e saúde"* [*"Analysis of the J48 and a priori mining algorithms applied to detect indicators of quality of life and health"*]. PhD diss. Universidade de Cruz Alta.
[24] Breiman, L. (2001). "Random Forests." *Machine Learning* 45(1): 5-32.
[25] Geurts, P., Ernst, D., and Wehenkel, L. (2006). "Extremely randomized trees." *Machine Learning* 63: 3-42.
[26] Landis, J. R., and Koch, G. G. (1977). "The measurement of observer agreement for categorical data." *Biometrics* 33(1): 159-174.
[27] Zhu, C., and Jiang, T. (2003). "Multicontext fuzzy clustering for separation of brain tissues in magnetic resonance images." *NeuroImage* 18: 685-696.

In: Understanding a Cancer Diagnosis
Editors: W. P. dos Santos et al.
ISBN: 978-1-53617-520-2
© 2020 Nova Science Publishers, Inc.

Chapter 6

METHOD FOR CLASSIFICATION OF BREAST LESIONS IN THERMOGRAPHIC IMAGES USING ELM CLASSIFIERS

Jessiane Mônica Silva Pereira[1],
Maíra Araújo de Santana[2],
Rita de Cássia Fernandes de Lima[3],
Sidney Marlon Lopes de Lima[4]
and Wellington Pinheiro dos Santos[2,*]

[1]Polytechnique School of the University of Pernambuco, Recife, Brazil
[2]Department of Biomedical Engineering, Federal University
of Pernambuco, Recife, Brazil
[3]Department of Mechanical Engineering, Federal University
of Pernambuco, Recife, Brazil
[4]Department of Electronics and Systems, Federal University
of Pernambuco, Recife, Brazil

---

* Corresponding Author's Email: wellington.santos@ufpe.br

ABSTRACT

This paper proposes a method to classify the type of breast lesion in thermographic images. The images were acquired at Hospital das Clínicas (HC) of Federal University of Pernambuco. They are from cases where there is a cyst, a malignant lesion or a benign lesion. Zernike and Haralick moments are used for extracting features based on shape and texture from these images. The Extreme Learning Machine (ELM) classifier was used to assess classification performance. Finally, the system performance is evaluated through the accuracy and Kappa statistic. From the use of the proposed method, the authors found an accuracy of 72.94% and 0.59 for Kappa statistic, which is considered moderate agreement between the expected and the obtained results.

Keywords: breast cancer, thermography, classification, ELM, Haralick, Zernike, breast lesion

INTRODUCTION

Breast cancer is the most common type of cancer among women. In Brazil, breast cancer mortality rates remain high due to the fact that the disease is still being diagnosed at advanced stages. Mammography is the most commonly used and indicated screening tool for breast cancer. This imaging method, however, is not as effective for women with dense, surgically altered breasts or those under 40 years of age. There is also some concern about the exposure to ionizing radiation and patient complaints about discomfort due to breast compression during mammography exam.

Breast thermography is being used as a complement to mammographic assessment. Thermography began to be used in mastology in 1959, but the lack of specialized professionals capable of understanding those images weakened the use of this method. With the advent of Computer Aided Diagnosis (CAD) systems, it was possible to further interpret those images, thus providing a more robust evaluation and a more accurate detection of breast alterations.

Many groups around the world are investing on CAD systems for breast cancer identification [1, 2, 3, 10, 11, 12, 13, 14]. Resmini et al. (2012) [1] perform several feature extractions and assess classification performances using each of the representations. They used SVM, kNN and Naïve Bayes as classifiers. In this study, the authors reach accuracy close to 90% and area below the ROC curve close to 0.9. Aguiar Junior et al. (2013) [2] also compared different ways to represent thermographic image using multilayer perceptron (MLP) as classifier. Their study achieved 75% of the correctly classified instances. Belfort, Silva and Paiva (2015) [3], perform feature extraction using Artificial Crawlers model. They used SVM to perform classification, founding 78% of accuracy, sensitivity of 50% and 84% specificity.

The main goal of the study presented in this chapter is to classify the type of breast lesion present in thermographic images. The authors used features extractors that provides an image representation based on texture and shape information. Finally, they tested several configuration of ELM classifier in an attempt to improve classification performance.

This chapter is organized as follows: first, the authors introduce the proposed method, then, they show and discuss their results and, finally, they present some conclusions and possible future approaches.

METHODS

In Figure 1 is the general fluxogram of the proposed method. The images used here are thermographic images that were acquired at Hospital das Clínicas (HC) from the Federal University of Pernambuco. These images were classified according to the type of lesion, so there are images where cyst is present, others show malignant lesion and others have benign lesion. For the preprocessing step, the RGB-JET image was converted to grayscale. A postprocessing step was performed to balance the classes. Zernike moments and Haralick moments are used for features. Finally, training is performed using different configuration of the Extreme Learning Machine.

The system performance is assessed through accuracy and Kappa statistic. These steps are further described below.

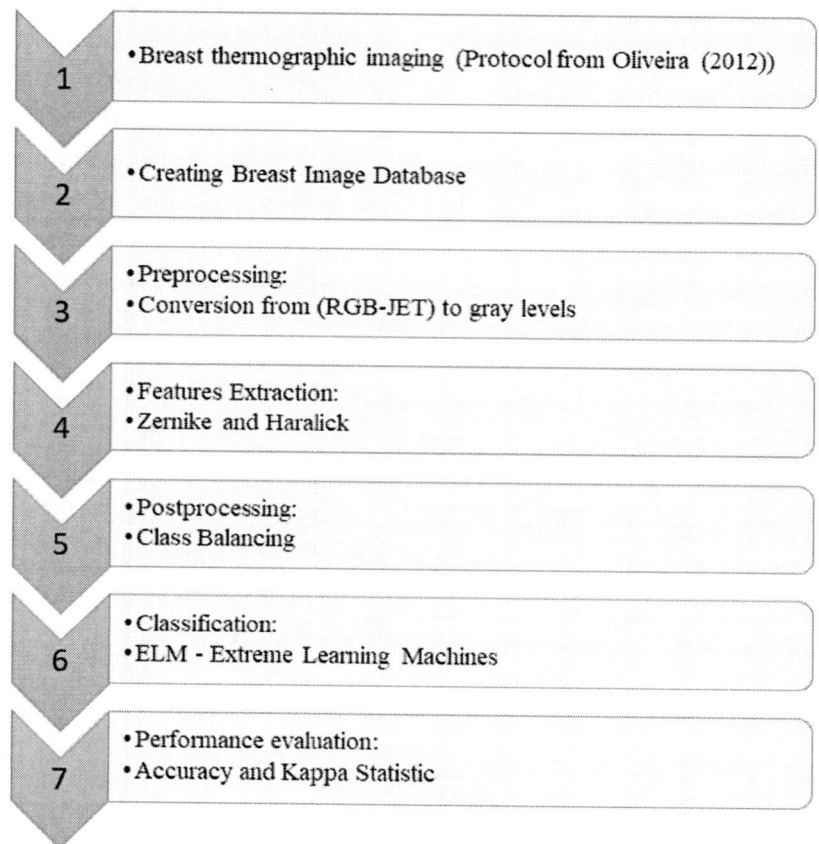

Source: The authors.

Figure 1. General fluxogram of the proposed method.

Image Acquisition

The thermographic images used in this study were acquired using a Flir S45 infrared camera and following the acquisition protocol defined by Oliveira (2012) [4]. According to Silva (2015) [5], the adopted method for the image acquisition was the static one. Eight images were acquired in each exam, each of these images are from different position. The first image is from the frontal view of both breasts with the hands on the waist (T1). The second image (T2), shows the frontal view of both breasts with raised hands holding a bar above the head. The third and fourth images are from frontal view of right and left breasts individually (MD and ME). They also acquired images from the inner and outer lateral views of each breast (LIMD, LIME, LEMD and LEME).

Creation of the Breast Thermographic Image Database

In this study the authors used the images in all the positions (T1, T2, MD, ME, LIMD, LIME, LEMD and LEME). Specialists previously diagnosed the image based on specific techniques for each clinical case [5]. The study in this chapter uses images where they found cyst, malignant lesion or benign lesion, so, each of these lesions represent a class in the problem present here. The Malignant Class comprises all biopsy-proven breast cancer cases. The Benign Class refers to cases of tumors with benignity, also confirmed by biopsy. The Cyst Class includes cases with this diagnosis proven by fine needle aspiration (FNA) or ultrasound [5].

Preprocessing

Thermographic images use pseudo-coloring technique, so each color actually represent a temperature. In this case, the images were acquired using the JET color palette. So, it was necessary to perform a conversion from RGB-JET to grayscale. This conversion was performed respecting the temperature information, in a way that the brighter spots represented the warmer regions and vice versa.

Features Extraction

The definition of the feature extraction method is one of the most important factors for the performance of a pattern recognition system [6]. So, for this study, the authors used Zernike moments to extract features related to shape or geometry and the Haralick moments to extract texture-based features. The first extractor creates projections of the image function into orthogonal base functions and is rotation invariant [7]. The second one calculates texture information based on the co-occurrence matrix from the image, assessing some characteristics of the gray level distribution along the image [6, 7].

Post Processing

After the features extraction, the authors performed a class balancing based on the linear balancing technique [14]. It was necessary because the database have different amount of images in each class.

Classification

For classification step, the extracted features were used as input to the classifier. So it is trained to learn each class features and patterns, and then, classify the images into one of the breast lesions classes (malignant, benign and cyst). In this chapter, the authors used the Extreme Learning Machine (ELM) as classifier. It is a training approach for single middle layer neural networks. This learning technique was proposed for training single hidden layer feedforward neural networks that accelerates learning by randomly generating input weights and hidden-layer biases [8].

In ELM, the hidden layer weights are randomly determined and have a nonlinear activation function while the output layer weights are analytically determined. Thus, ELM has a simple implementation and temporal reduction [8].

The training was conducted using two test modes. The first one was using 66% of the database for training and the remaining for test. Then, the authors used 75% of the database for training. The authors also tested different configurations of ELM by changing the number of neurons in the hidden layer and the kernel function. They used 100, 200, 300, 400 and 500 neurons and using linear kernel and polynomial kernel with exponents (p) of 2, 3, 4 and 5.

Performance Evaluation

Finally, the system performance was evaluated through the accuracy and Kappa statistic. Accuracy is a percentage of correctly classified data [9]. Kappa statistic is a statistical method for assessing the level of agreement or reproducibility between the expected and the obtained results, it may assume values from -1 to 1 (see Table 1 for further information) [9].

Table 1. Meaning of Kappa statistic values

Kappa values	Concordance
<0	None
0-0.20	Weak
0.21-0.40	Considerable
0.41-0.60	Moderate
0.61-0.80	Substantial
0.81-1.0	Great

RESULTS AND DISCUSSION

As mentioned before, the authors used accuracy and Kappa statistical to assess classification performance. Figures 2 to 7 show the results of the classification accuracy (in (a)) and kappa statistic (in (b)) for the datasets using Haralick, Zernike and Haralick and Zernike features extraction method, for both test modes (with 66% and 75% of the base).

Figures 2 and 3 show ELM performance for the dataset using only Haralick features to represent the thermographic images. The results in Figure 2 were achieved when using 66% of the database for training, while Figure 3 shows the results using 75% of the database.

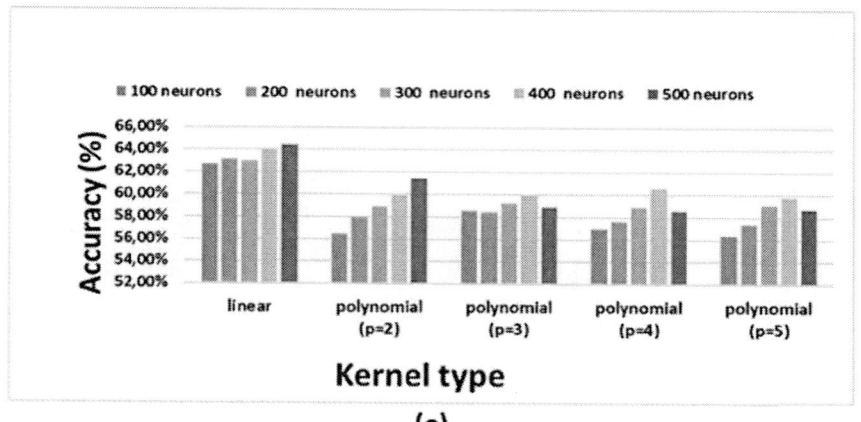

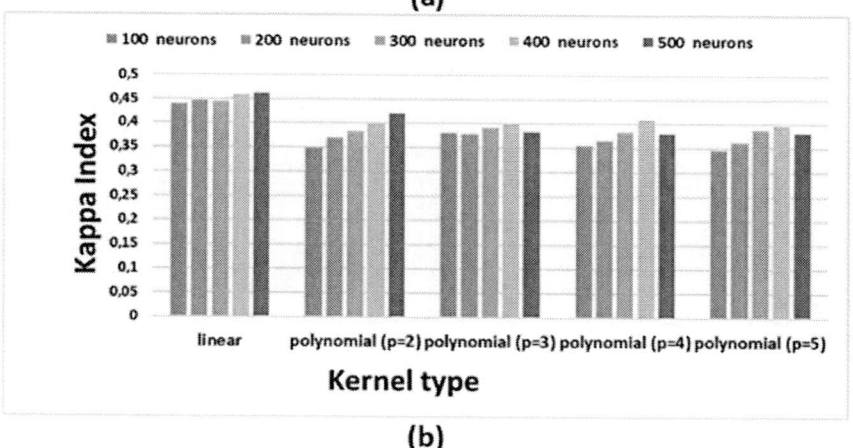

Source: The authors.

Figure 2. Results of (a) accuracy and (b) kappa statistic when using the features from Haralick moments and 66% of the database for training.

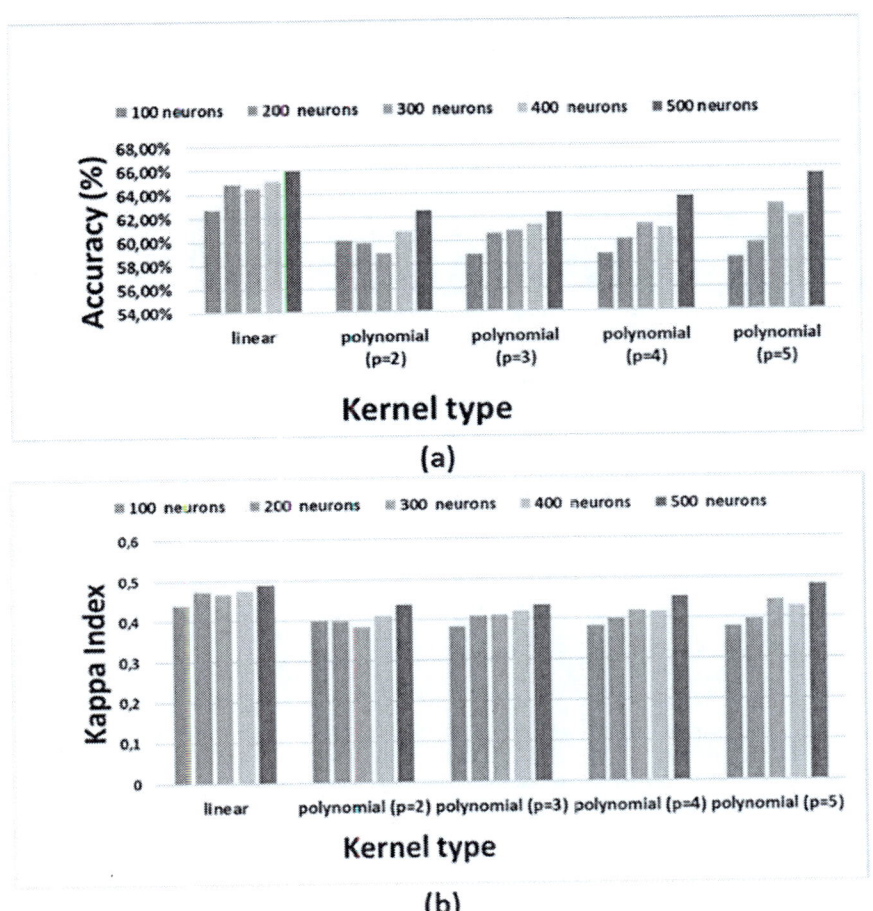

Source: The authors.

Figure 3. Results of (a) accuracy and (b) kappa statistic when using the features from Haralick moments and 75% of the database for training.

Figure 4 shows ELM performance for the dataset using only features extracted using Zernike moments and using 66% of the database for training and the remaining for test. The results using 75% of the database and Zernike features alone are shown in Figure 5.

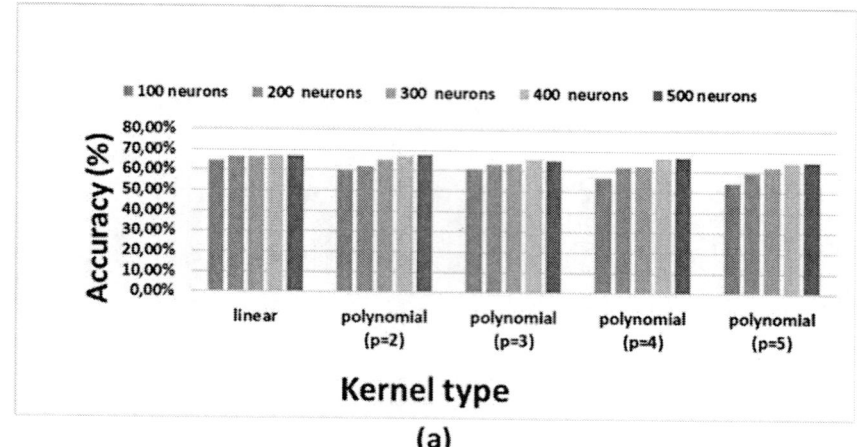

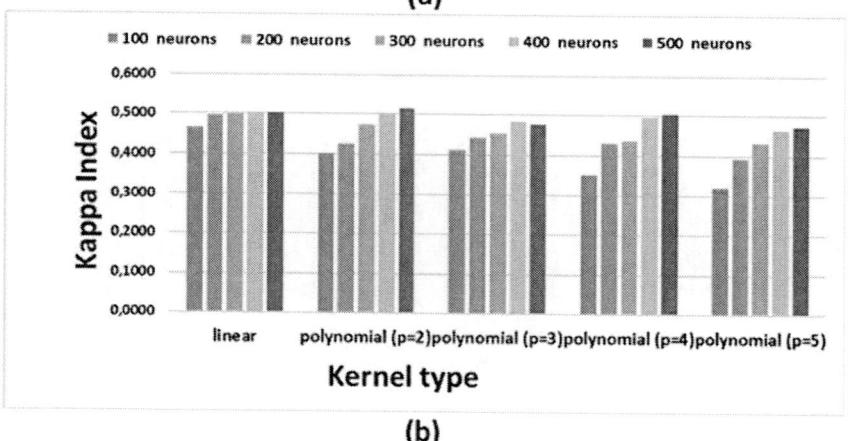

Source: The authors.

Figure 4. Results of (a) accuracy and (b) kappa statistic when using the features from Zernike moments and 66% of the database for training.

Figures 6 and 7 present ELM performance when the authors combined the features from Haralick and Zernike moments and used, respectively, 66% and 75% of the database for training.

From Figures 2 to 7, the authors verified that the configuration that presented better results was when using 500 neurons in the hidden layer, linear kernel and the combination of Haralick and Zernike features.

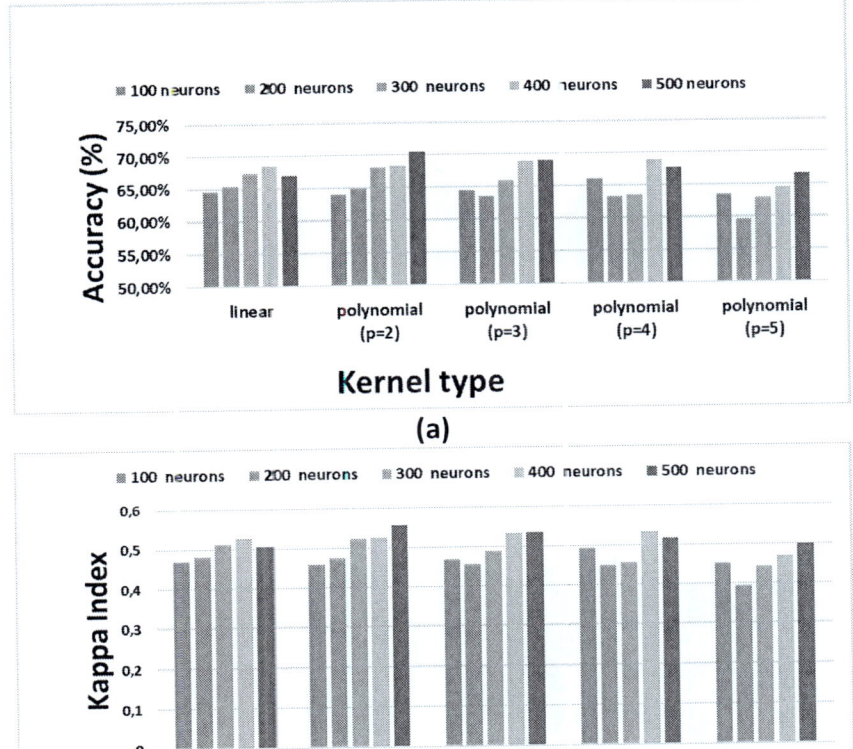

Source: The authors.

Figure 5. Results of (a) accuracy and (b) kappa statistic when using the features from Zernike moments and 75% of the database for training.

Regarding to the test mode, the results were very similar when using both configurations (66% or 75%), however, slightly better results were found when splitting the database in 75% for training and the remaining for test. The best result overall was an accuracy of 72.94%, with a kappa statistic of 0.59 (Figure 7).

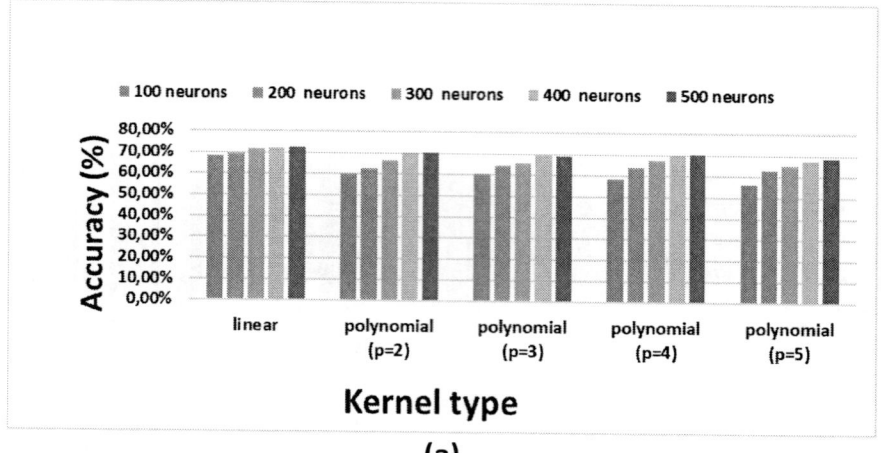

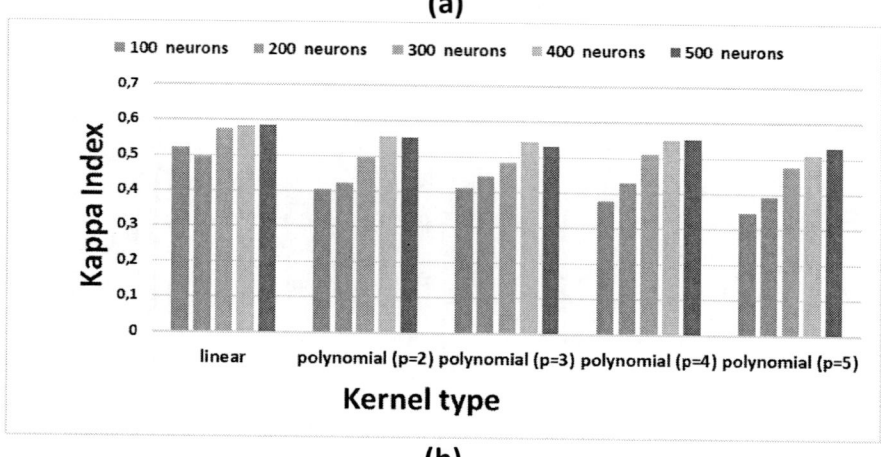

Source: The authors.

Figure 6. Results of (a) accuracy and (b) kappa statistic when using the features from both Haralick and Zernike moments and 66% of the database for training.

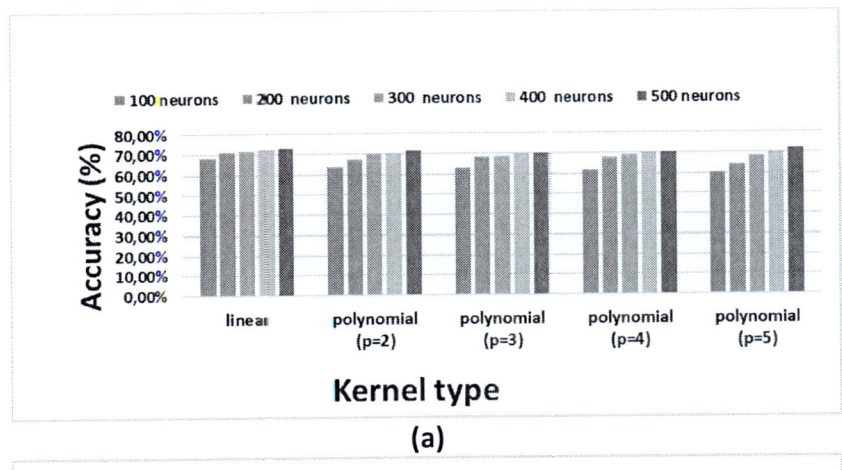

(a)

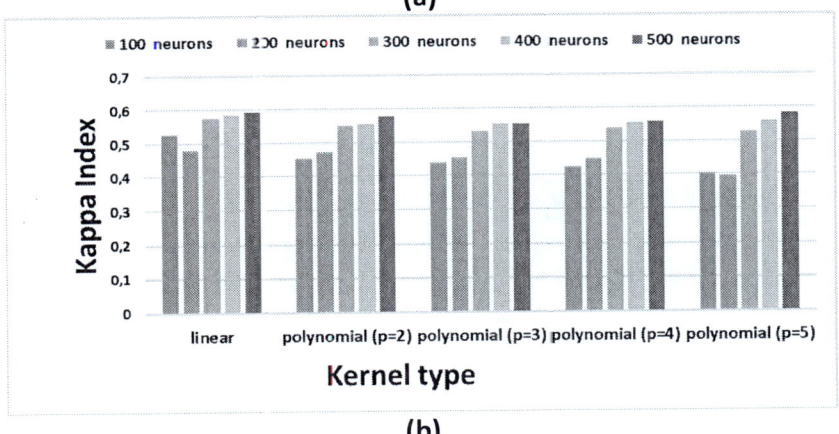

(b)

Source: The authors.

Figure 7. Results of (a) accuracy and (b) kappa statistic when using the features from both Haralick and Zernike moments and 75% of the database for training.

CONCLUSION

This chapter presented a proposal for a breast lesion classification method using geometry-based (Zernike moments) and texture-based (Haralick moments) features extractors and their combination. The authors performed experiments using different configurations of ELM classifier, in order to assess its best performance.

Table 2. Best results using ELM classifier and Haralick, Zernike and the combination of Haralick and Zernike descriptors

Configuration	Accuracy (%)	Kappa Statistic
Haralick features extractor, 500 neurons, linear kernel and training using 66% of database.	64.42	0.4623
Haralick features extractor, 500 neurons, linear kernel and training using 75% of database.	65.95%	0.4892
Zernike features extractor, 500 neurons, linear kernel and training using 66% of database.	67.72%	0.5158
Zernike features extractor, 500 neurons, linear kernel and training using 75% of the database.	70.43%	0.5564
Haralick and Zernike features extractors, 500 neurons, linear kernel and training using 66% of the database.	72.22%	0.5833
Haralick and Zernike features extractors, 500 neurons, linear kernel and training using 75% of the database.	72.94%	0.5940

As previously seen, the ELM classifier achieved its best performance when the images were represented by the combination of the features extracted from Zernike and Haralick methods. It shows that both shape and texture information are important to differentiate breast lesions in thermographic images.

Regarding to ELM configuration, the linear kernel provided the best results when combined to 500 neurons in the hidden layer. For the training mode, the results were very similar when changing the training mode, but slightly better results were found by using 75% of the database for training.

Overall, the method achieved accuracy up to 72.94% and Kappa statistic of 0.59, which is considered moderate agreement between the obtained result and the expected result.

For future studies, the authors may invest on the assessment of other classifiers, including deep learning approaches. Features selection studies may also be performed to improve system efficiency.

ACKNOWLEDGMENTS

We thank FACEPE, CAPES and CNPq for their financial support.

REFERENCES

[1] Resmini, R., Conci, A., Borchartt, T. B., Lima, R. C. F., Montenegro, A. A., and Pantaleão, C. A. (2012). "Diagnóstico Precoce de Doenças Mamárias Usando Imagens Térmicas e Aprendizado de Máquina" ["Early Diagnosis of Breast Diseases Using Thermal Imaging and Machine Learning."] *Revista Eletrônica do Alto Vale do Itajaí* 1(1): 55-67.

[2] Aguiar Junior, P. S., Belfort, C. N. S., Silva, A. C., Diniz, P. H. B., Lima, R. C. F., Conci, A., and Paiva, A. C. (2013). "Detecção de Regiões Suspeitas de Lesão na Mama em Imagens Térmicas Utilizando Spatiogram e Redes Neurais." ["Detection of Suspected Breast Injury Regions in Thermal Imaging Using Spatiogram and Neural Networks."] *Cadernos de Pesquisa* 20(2):56-63.

[3] Belfort, C. N. S., Silva, A. C., and Paiva, A. C. (2015). "Detecção de lesões em imagens termográficas de mama utilizando Índice de Similaridade de Jaccard e Artificial Crawlers" ["Lesion detection in breast thermographic images using Jaccard Similarity Index and Artificial Crawlers"] Paper presented at the *XV Workshop de Informática Médica*, Recife, Brazil.

[4] Oliveira, M. M. (2012). "Desenvolvimento de protocolo e construção de um aparato mecânico para padronização da aquisição de imagens termográficas de mama" ["Protocol development and construction of a mechanical apparatus for standardization of breast thermographic imaging"] Master's thesis, Federal University of Pernambuco.

[5] Silva, A. S. V. (2015). "Classificação e segmentação de termogramas de mama para triagem de pacientes residentes em regiões de poucos recursos médicos" ["Classification and segmentation of breast

thermograms for screening patients residing in low-resource regions."] Master's thesis, Federal University of Pernambuco, Brazil.

[6] Cheng, H. D., Shi, X. J., Min, R., Hu, L. M., Cai, X. P., and Du, H. N. (2006). "Approaches for automated detection and classification of masses in mammograms." *Pattern Recognition* 39(4): 646-668.

[7] Shanthi, S., and Bhaskaran, V. M. (2013). "A Novel Approach for Detecting and Classifying Breast Cancer in Mammogram Images." *International Journal of Intelligent Information Technologies (IJIIT)*, 9(1): 21-39.

[8] Huang, G. B., Zhu, Q. Y., and Siew C. K. (2006). "Extreme learning machine: Theory and applications." *Neurocomputing* 70(1): 489-501. ISSN 09252312.

[9] Ladis, R. J., and Koch, G. G. (1977). "The Measurement of Observer Agreement for Categorical Data." *Biometrics* 33: 159-174.

[10] Acharya, U. R., Ng, E. Y. K., Tan, J. H., and Sree, S. V. (2012). "Thermography Based Breast Cancer Detection Using Texture Features and Support Vector Machine." *Journal of Medical Systems* 36(3):1503-10.

[11] Azevedo, W. W., Lima, S. M. L., Fernandes, I. M. M., Rocha, A. D. D., Cordeiro, F. R., Silva-Filho, A. G., and Santos, W. P. (2015). "Morphological extreme learning machines applied to detect and classify masses in mammograms" Paper presented at *2015 International Joint Conference of Neural Networks (IJCNN)*, Killarney, Ireland.

[12] Rodrigues, A. L., Santana, M. A., Azevedo, W. W., Bezerra, R. S., Santos, W. P., and Lima, R. C. F. (2018). "Seleção de Atributos para Apoio ao Diagnóstico do Câncer de Mama Usando Imagens Termográficas, Algoritmos Genéticos e Otimização por Enxame de Partículas" ["Feature Selection to Support Breast Cancer Diagnosis Using Thermographic Imaging, Genetic Algorithms, and Particle Swarm Optimization"] Paper presented at *II Simpósio de Inovação em Engenharia Biomédica (SABIO 2018)*, Recife, Brazil.

[13] Santana, M. A., Pereira, J. M. S., Silva, F. L., Lima, N. M., Sousa, F. N., Arruda, G. M. S., Lima, R. C. F., Silva, W. W. A., and Santos, W.

P. (2018). "Breast cancer diagnosis based on mammary thermography and extreme learning machines." *Research on Biomedical Engineering* 34(1):45-53. Epub March 05, 2018. https://dx.doi.org/ 10.1590/2446-4740.05217.

[14] Lima, S. M. L, Silva-Filho, A. G., and Santos, W. P. (2016). "Detection and classification of masses in mammographic images in a multi-kernel approach." *Computer Methods and Programs in Biomedicine* 134:11-29. doi: 10.1016/j.cmpb.2016.04.029.

ABOUT THE EDITORS

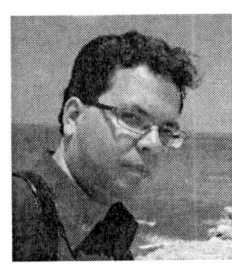

Prof. Wellington Pinheiro dos Santos is an Associate Professor at the Department of Biomedical Engineering of the Federal University of Pernambuco, Recife, Brazil. He received his BSc and MSc in Electrical Engineering at UFPE, Brazil, and his PhD in Electrical Engineering from the Federal University of Campina Grande, Brazil, in 2009. He is interested in how early diagnosis based on signals and images could be improved by using Artificial Intelligence, especially in diseases like breast cancer and Alzheimer's. His main research interests are applied artificial intelligence in health, artificial neural networks, evolutionary computation, image diagnosis, computer-aided diagnostic systems, applied neuroscience, serious games, and innovation in health.

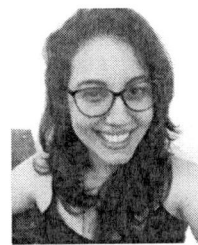

Maíra Araújo de Santana is an assistant researcher at the Department of Biomedical Engineering of the Federal University of Pernambuco, Recife, Brazil. She is graduated in Biomedical Engineering. She received her BSc and MSc in Biomedical Engineering from the Federal University of Pernambuco, Brazil. Maíra is very interested in how we could understand breast cancer dynamics and how Artificial Intelligence could help us to get earlier and more accurate diagnostics. She is also interested in applied neuroscience, studying rehabilitation engineering and the effects of music in children and elderly people.

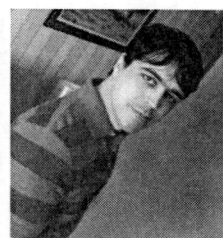

Dr. Washington Wagner Azevedo da Silva is a post-doctoral researcher at the Department of Biomedical Engineering of the Federal University of Pernambuco, Recife, Brazil. He received his PhD in Computer Science from the Federal University of Pernambuco, Brazil, his MSc in Computer Science at UFPE, Brazil and BSc in Systems Analysis at UNIVERSO, Brazil.

He works on neural networks architectures to improve image analysis and processing. His principal research themes are computer-aided diagnosis, kernel-based classifiers and artificial intelligence in health.

INDEX

A

androgen receptor (AR) inhibitors, 2, 3, 4, 6, 7, 10, 11, 20, 21, 23
androgen signaling, 10
antibody, 6, 7, 9, 20
antitumor, 7, 9
artificial neural networks, 57, 74, 157, 123

B

benign lesion, ix, 33, 36, 37, 77, 82, 83, 85, 86, 87, 96, 98, 125, 140, 141, 143
biomarkers, 9, 11, 20, 21
biopsy, 42, 77, 94, 96, 125, 143
blood flow, 75, 93
BRCA1, 2, 3, 5, 8, 9, 16, 17, 18, 19, 20, 21, 22, 23, 25
BRCA1/2 mutation, 2, 5, 8, 18, 20
BRCA2, 2, 3, 5, 16, 19, 22, 25
BRCAness, 5, 23
BRCA-proficient, 5
breast cancer (BC), vi, viii, ix, x, xi, 1, 2, 3, 4, 5, 6, 7, 8, 10, 12, 13, 14, 15, 16, 17, 18, 19, 20, 21, 22, 23, 24, 25, 27, 28, 29, 30, 31, 32, 33, 53, 57, 65, 66, 68, 71, 72, 74, 88, 89, 92, 94, 105, 106, 107, 111, 112, 113, 115, 134, 135, 137, 140, 141, 143, 154, 157, 158
breast lesion, ix, 29, 52, 60, 74, 75, 77, 81, 87, 92, 93, 104, 112, 113, 115, 128, 134, 140, 141, 144, 151, 152
breast mass, 35, 40, 41, 55, 56, 63
breast thermography, ix, 74, 76, 92, 93, 97, 134

C

CAD, ix, 140, 141
cancer, vii, viii, ix, x, 2, 4, 7, 12, 14, 16, 18, 19, 20, 22, 25, 27, 28, 29, 30, 31, 33, 35, 36, 64, 65, 70, 74, 75, 92, 94, 106, 107, 112, 113, 115, 135, 140, 155
cancer cells, 20, 75, 112
cancer death, 27, 28, 92, 113
CD8+, 8
checkpoint inhibitors, 2, 6, 20, 21
chemotherapy, 3, 4, 7, 14, 23, 24
clinical trials, 2, 6, 10, 12, 13, 20

Index

computer-aided diagnosis (CAD), ix, 140, 141, 158
cyst, 77, 82, 83, 85, 86, 96, 98, 125, 128, 140, 141, 143, 144

D

death rate, 29, 31
deaths, 29, 30, 31, 74
decomposition, 28, 33, 38, 47, 48, 53, 55, 56
detection, ix, x, 29, 34, 35, 36, 51, 52, 54, 55, 57, 63, 65, 68, 69, 74, 75, 89, 92, 93, 94, 102, 104, 107, 112, 113, 115, 134, 137, 140, 153, 154
developed countries, 30, 31
developing countries, viii, 29, 30, 31

E

early diagnosis, 92, 113, 157
Extreme Learning Machine (ELM), vi, ix, 28, 33, 51, 57, 58, 59, 70, 71, 74, 75, 78, 79, 80, 81, 82, 86, 87, 88, 89, 107, 112, 114, 122, 124, 128, 131, 134, 135, 139, 140, 141, 144, 145, 146, 147, 148, 151, 152, 154, 155

F

false negative, 104, 105, 113
false positive, 104
feature selection, 114, 128, 131, 134
features extraction, 77, 78, 92, 95, 96, 100, 102, 103, 144, 145
features selection, ix, 94, 105, 112, 114, 115, 119, 127, 128, 131, 134

G

gene expression, 11
gene promoter, 5
genes, 3, 5, 9, 94
genetic mutations, 16
genetic testing, 14, 16, 17, 18
growth factor, 2, 3, 4, 7

H

Haralick, v, ix, 73, 74, 77, 78, 79, 80, 81, 82, 83, 85, 86, 90, 92, 93, 100, 102, 103, 104, 106, 108, 114, 127, 130, 140, 141, 144, 145, 146, 147, 148, 150, 151, 152
Haralick moments, 74, 77, 78, 79, 82, 83, 92, 100, 102, 104, 105, 114, 127, 140, 141, 144, 146, 147, 151
Haralick moments and Zernike moments, 77, 82, 92, 100, 105, 114
hegemony, 118, 121, 122

I

image analysis, 42, 69, 95, 106
immunohistochemistry, 7, 10
immunotherapy, 2, 3, 9, 20, 21
intervention, 32, 34, 35, 36, 37, 38, 54
ionizing radiation, 75, 92, 93, 113, 115, 140

L

learning machine, 68, 70, 74, 135, 154
lesions, ix, 28, 29, 30, 32, 34, 35, 36, 37, 38, 41, 42, 43, 51, 55, 60, 64, 71, 74, 75, 77, 79, 85, 86, 87, 92, 93, 104, 112, 113, 115, 128, 134, 136, 143, 144, 152

M

machine learning, ix, xi, 92, 93, 94, 109, 115, 127
magnetic resonance imaging (MRI), 19, 69, 92, 113, 115
malignant lesion, 33, 34, 43, 52, 55, 57, 64, 77, 82, 83, 86, 87, 96, 98, 125, 140, 141, 143
malignant tumors, 41
mammogram, 38, 69
mammography, 19, 28, 32, 34, 35, 38, 41, 46, 53, 63, 68, 77, 92, 93, 96, 106, 112, 113, 115, 136, 140
mastectomy, 19, 29
mathematical morphology, 28
morphological decomposition, 28
morphology, 28, 56, 69
mortality rate, viii, 27, 29, 30, 65, 74, 92,
mutation, 2, 3, 5, 6, 7, 8, 9, 16, 17, 18, 19, 20, 22, 23, 117

N

neural networks, 36, 57, 58, 63, 74, 114, 124, 131, 144
neurons, 36, 51, 57, 58, 78, 79, 81, 124, 129, 145, 148, 152
no lesion, 28, 57, 96, 98, 99, 125, 128

O

obesity, 28, 29, 31, 66
ODM, ix, 112, 114, 116, 127, 128, 131, 134
OECD, 66
oophorectomy, 19
operations, 33, 45, 53, 55
optimization, ix, 70, 112, 114, 116, 117, 119, 120, 122, 123, 125, 127, 134, 136
optimization and classification, 112

optimization method, 117, 122, 123, 125
ovarian cancer, 17, 22, 25

P

paclitaxel, 6, 7, 8, 11, 23, 24
parenchyma, 39, 40, 41, 43
poly(ADP-ribose) polymerase (PARP) inhibitors, 2, 3, 5, 6, 7, 8, 14, 16, 17, 18, 20, 21
polymerase, 2, 3, 5, 7, 14, 17
progesterone, 2, 3, 7
prognosis, 3, 10, 74, 115
programmed cell death ligand 1 (PD-L1), 2, 6, 7, 8, 9, 20, 21, 24
programmed cell death protein-1 (PD-1), 2, 6, 7, 9, 20

Q

quality of life, 1, 2, 3, 138

R

radiation, 7, 14, 75, 92, 106, 113, 115
radiation therapy, 7, 14
radiotherapy, 9
ribose, 2, 3, 5, 7, 14, 17

S

stem cells, 22
survival, 7, 9, 10, 20, 21, 23
synthesis, 117, 119, 121, 122

T

targeted therapy, 2, 13, 14, 18, 19, 20, 25
techniques, x, 10, 32, 35, 61, 62, 74, 75, 94, 95, 100, 106, 112, 113, 123, 127, 143

Index

therapy, 2, 7, 8, 9, 11, 12, 13, 14, 18, 19, 20, 23, 25
thermograms, 95, 108, 137, 154
thermography, ix, 70, 74, 76, 89, 92, 93, 94, 97, 105, 106, 107, 112, 113, 134, 135, 140, 155
thermoregulation, 93
Triple-Negative Breast Cancer (TNBC), v, viii, 2, 3, 4, 5, 6, 7, 8, 9, 10, 11, 12, 13, 15, 16, 20, 21, 22, 23, 24, 25
tumor, 5, 6, 8, 9, 10, 13, 16, 20, 21, 46, 68, 93, 95, 106, 112, 125, 143

U

ultrasonography, 92, 96, 113
ultrasound, 77, 115, 125, 143

V

vascularization, 93

W

wavelet analysis, 68
wavelet(s), ix, 28, 33, 38, 46, 47, 48, 53, 56, 59, 60, 62, 68, 136
World Health Organization (WHO), 27, 66, 74, 88, 92

X

x-rays, 93

Y

young women, 12, 39, 113

Z

Zernike, v, ix, 33, 35, 37, 49, 50, 56, 57, 71, 73, 74, 77, 78, 79, 80, 81, 82, 84, 85, 86, 90, 92, 93, 100, 102, 103, 104, 106, 108, 114, 127, 130, 140, 141, 144, 145, 147, 148, 149, 150, 151, 152
Zernike moments, 33, 35, 37, 49, 56, 57, 74, 77, 78, 79, 82, 84, 85, 86, 92, 100, 102, 103, 104, 106, 108, 114, 127, 130, 141, 144, 147, 148, 149, 150, 151